Praise and Endorsements

I am thrilled to see this book by Dr. Steven D. Roffers, DC. I have known Steven for more than 20 years. We first met as fellow chiropractic students, and he even attended my wedding to Tricia Carrick-Antonucci. Over the years, he has become not only a trusted friend but also a valued colleague. Dr. Roffers and I frequently discuss a wide range of issues affecting the chiropractic profession, and I am continually grateful for his wisdom, experience, and thoughtful perspective. Whether you are a patient seeking to better understand your health, a chiropractor looking to deepen your appreciation for the profession, or simply someone interested in how the body functions and heals, you will find this book informative, engaging, and inspiring. *—Dr. Matthew M. Antonucci, DC, DACNB, FACFN, FICC; Board-Certified Chiropractic Neurologist, Researcher, and International Lecturer*

In **Life Is Better Adjusted**, Dr. Steven Roffers, DC delivers a clear, practical, and evidence-informed explanation of what chiropractic is, how it works, and why it deserves a place in modern healthcare. I've known Steven for more than 11 years now, and throughout that time I've been consistently impressed by his passion, integrity, and commitment to improving patient care. I had the privilege of participating in three chiropractic research studies with him, each contributing to the growing body of scientific evidence supporting conservative care. In this book, Dr. Roffers thoughtfully explains not only the role of chiropractic but also the importance of physical therapy, nutrition, movement, and healthy lifestyle habits in creating the environment the body needs to heal and thrive. Whether you're a patient, healthcare professional, or simply someone who wants to better understand how the body functions, this book is an outstanding resource. *—Dr. J. Michael Menke, DC, PhD; Independent Researcher, University of Arizona School of Mind, Brain, and Behavior*

I was Steven's Faculty Advisor at Life University's Outpatient Clinic. I was so happy, proud, and honored when he received the "Clinic Excellence Award" while he was a student. I knew there was something special about Steven! I am not surprised by his accomplishments which also include publication of this book. **Life Is Better Adjusted** is a comprehensive look at chiropractic, and its application, and how everyone can benefit. *—Dr. Milagros Rosado, DC; Atabey Quiropraxia*

If you've been doing everything you know to improve your health yet still don't feel your best, this book offers a refreshing and insightful perspective. Dr. Steven Roffers, DC is one of the most compassionate and knowledgeable healthcare professionals I have ever encountered. In this book, he combines clinical expertise with a gift for making complex concepts easy to understand. The result is a powerful guide that helps readers better understand the incredible design of the human body and the important role chiropractic care can play in restoring health and vitality. *—Cynthia Loy Darst, Master Certified Coach; Team Darst*

Life Is Better Adjusted

How Chiropractic "Works" and Why Everyone Can Benefit From It

DR. STEVEN D. ROFFERS, DC

ISBN - Paperback: 9798997881801

ISBN - Hardcover: 9798997881818

Disclaimer

The content provided in this book is designed to provide helpful information on the subjects discussed. This book is not meant to be used, nor should it be used, to diagnose or treat any medical condition. The publisher and the authors are not responsible for any actions you take or do not take as a result of reading this book.

Dedication and Appreciation

Dedication

I dedicate this book to my mom, Jacqueline Mary VanDenBusch (December 17, 1935 to October 25, 2021). My mom was the best teacher ever… Every time I asked her "Why?" she would respond with the best education. Every time I pestered her with my incessant "So?" she would reply with the best explanations… until she'd reply with "Sew buttons on your underwear" and then I knew I better stop! If you know, you know.

Appreciation

I have so many people to thank for helping me make this book a reality. First and foremost, I thank Ivan Da Silva, my husband and the most amazing life partner in every sense of that term. I will thank others personally.

Table of Contents

Introduction

✦✦✦

Your Body Is Talking — Are You Listening?

Something is happening inside your body right now that you probably cannot feel yet.

Your spine is changing. Your discs are shifting. The nerves that carry signals from your brain to every single organ, muscle, and cell in your body are either flowing freely or getting squeezed or impeded. The direction all of this is moving in isn't random. It is not bad luck. It is not just "getting older." It is a process that follows a very specific set of rules, and once you understand those rules, you can actually do something about them.

Most people don't pick up a book like this until something hurts. They wait until the pain gets bad enough that ignoring it stops being an option. And that's understandable. Life is busy. You've got work, family, responsibilities, and a hundred other things pulling your attention in every direction. The body gets put on the back burner until it forces its way to the front.

But you picked this up.

That matters more than you might think. Because the people who make real, lasting changes to their health aren't the ones who waited until everything fell apart. They are the ones who got curious before the crisis hit. They are the ones who asked, "why is this happening?" instead of just reaching for the ibuprofen and hoping for the best. If that sounds like you, you're in exactly the right place. Welcome!

There is a force working against your body every single day. It doesn't care how old you are, how fit you are, or how well you eat. It works on everyone, all the time, without exception. Scientists call it "entropy," and it's the same force that rusts metal, crumbles old buildings, and turns a clean room into a mess the moment you stop tidying it. Left unchecked, it moves everything from order to disorder. And your body is not exempt from that rule.

The good news is that entropy is not a death sentence. It is a Universal Law you can work with once you understand it. And that's exactly what this book is going to show you how to do.

Think about a hypothetical person for a moment. Let's call her Maria, a 52-year-old school administrator who has been waking up stiff every morning for the past three years. Her lower back aches by midday. Her neck is tight by evening. She has been told by her doctor that everything "looks fine" on her bloodwork and that the aches are "just part of aging." So, she stretches a little, takes something for the pain when it gets bad, and keeps moving. She figures this is just what 52 feels like. What Maria doesn't know is that her body has been sending her signals for years, and the stiffness she feels every morning isn't just aging. It is a warning! Her spine has been slowly losing the battle against entropy, and the pain she's experiencing now is not the beginning of the problem. It is nearing the late-stage signal of something that started long before she ever noticed it.

Maria's story isn't unusual. It is actually the norm. And if any part of it sounds familiar to you, this book was written with you in mind.

Your body is always moving in one direction or the other. Toward health or toward breakdown. There is no standing still, no pause button, no neutral gear. Every single day, the choices you make, the way you sit, the way you move, the care you give your spine and nervous system, are either pushing back against entropy or letting it win a little more ground. That is not meant to scare you. It is meant to wake you up, and get your attention, because once you understand that you stop being a passenger (passive) in your own health and start being the driver (active).

Pain is not the problem. Pain is the alarm that goes off after the problem has already been building for months, sometimes years. Waiting for pain before you take action is like waiting for your house to catch fire before you check whether the smoke detector works. By the time the alarm sounds, a lot of damage has already been done. This book is going to change the way you think about pain, about your spine, and about what it actually means to be healthy.

You don't have to be in crisis to benefit from what's in these pages. Whether you're dealing with serious, daily pain or just that low-level stiffness and fatigue that you've quietly accepted as normal, this book has something for you. And if you're someone who feels fairly good right now and wants to stay that way for the next thirty or forty years, this book especially has something for you.

What You'll Learn and Why This Book Is Different

There's no shortage of health books out there. Stretch more. Drink more water. Sleep eight hours. Eat your vegetables. Take this supplement. Take that vitamin. See your doctor. You've heard it all before, and while none of that advice is wrong exactly, it is missing something critical. It doesn't explain the underlying reason your body breaks down in the first place. It gives you tips without giving you the framework that makes those tips make sense.

This book is built differently.

What you're going to get here is the missing piece. The explanation that connects the dots between why your back or neck hurts, why your energy is low, why you feel older than you really are, and what one specific system in your body controls all of it. That system is your nervous system. And the structure that protects it, the structure that either keeps it running at full power or slowly chokes it off, is your spine.

Most health conversations completely skip over the nervous system. They talk about muscles, joints, inflammation, and diet. All of those things matter. But the nervous system is the Master Controller. It runs every function in your body, from your heartbeat to your digestion to your immune response to the way your muscles fire when you move. And when the spine that houses and protects it starts to break down, the effects ripple out into every corner of your health in ways that most people never connect back to their spine.

You are going to learn why pain is actually a terrible yet important warning system. You are going to understand why spinal degeneration starts silently, often decades before you feel anything, and why that changes everything about how you should think about prevention. You are going to learn about something called "innate intelligence," which is your body's built-in ability to heal and regulate itself when the nervous system is free from interference. And you are going to understand why most conventional health advice treats the symptom while completely ignoring the root cause.

This book also addresses something that almost nobody talks about in the context of spinal health, and that's performance and function. Most people think chiropractic care is for people who are already in pain. That's like saying a gym is only for people who are already out of shape. Spinal health and nervous system function are just as important for the athlete who wants to perform at their best as they are for the person who can barely get out of bed in the morning. The two goals are not separate. They are the same goal at different points on the same scale.

You will not find vague advice in these pages. Every concept comes with a clear explanation of why it matters and what you can actually do about it. The goal isn't to impress you with science. The goal is to hand you a clear, honest, actionable picture of what is happening inside your body and give you the tools to change it starting today.

The Road Map — Here's Where We're Going

Before you get into the heart of this book, it helps to know where you are headed. Here is a clear look at the ground we are going to cover together.

We start with "entropy" itself. We define and describe in detail what entropy is, why your body isn't exempt from it, and how this one concept reframes everything you think you know about aging and physical decline. This is the foundation that everything else in the book is built on, and it's the idea you will keep coming back to no matter where you are in your health right now.

From there, we move into the spine. You'll learn what spinal degeneration actually looks like at the structural level, how it starts long before you feel it, and why the common assumption that "if it doesn't hurt, it's fine" is one of the most expensive mistakes a person can make with their health. You will understand what is actually happening inside your discs, your vertebrae, and the spaces where your nerves travel, and why keeping those structures healthy is about so much more than avoiding back pain.

Then we get into the nervous system, and this is where things start to get genuinely eye-opening. You will learn how the spine and the nervous system are connected, why a healthy spine means a fully functioning nervous system, and what happens to your entire body when that connection gets compromised. You will understand the difference between your sympathetic and parasympathetic nervous systems, why chronic stress and poor spinal health can lock your body into a constant state of tension and dysfunction, and what it takes to shift out of that state and into one where healing and recovery can actually happen.

We will cover a brief history of chiropractic care because context matters. Understanding where this field came from, how it developed, and what the science actually says gives you a much clearer picture of why spinal manipulation is a legitimate, well-studied, and powerful tool for restoring function. It also helps you cut through the noise of skepticism and misinformation that still surrounds chiropractic care in some circles.

The concept of innate intelligence gets its own deep look. Your body already knows how to heal. It has been doing it your entire life, every time you have cut your finger, fought off a cold, or recovered from an injury. The question is not whether your body can heal. The question is whether it has the clear neurological pathways it needs to do that job properly. Spinal health is what keeps those pathways open.

We will also spend real time on what return to function actually looks like in practice. Return to work. Return to play. Return to the activities that make your life feel like yours again. These aren't just feel-good ideas. They are measurable, achievable outcomes that come from taking spinal health seriously, and they apply whether you're a 28-year-old athlete recovering from an injury or a 68-year-old retiree who wants to keep hiking on the weekends.

By the time you reach the final pages, you will have a complete picture. You'll understand why your body breaks down, what system controls the whole thing, and exactly what steps you can take to slow the breakdown, reverse damage that's already been done, and build a foundation of health that actually holds up over time. Not just less pain! More life. More energy. More function. More of the moments that matter.

That is the real promise of this book. Not a quick fix. Not a miracle cure. A clear, honest, science-backed explanation of what is happening inside your body, paired with a practical roadmap for doing something about it. The kind of roadmap that makes you feel like you finally understand what has been going on, and more importantly, what you can actually do about it starting right now.

Your body has been talking to you for a long time. This book teaches you how to listen, and how to answer back.

Entropy — The Silent Force That's Been Working Against You

✦✦✦

What Entropy Actually Is and Why Your Body Isn't Exempt

Your car doesn't stay clean on its own. Your house doesn't stay organized without effort. Left alone long enough, everything around you slowly falls apart, breaks down, and moves toward disorder. This isn't bad luck. It is physics. Actually, it's more specifically thermodynamics. The same force that rusts your car, crumbles old buildings, and turns a tidy room into chaos is working on your body right now, whether you feel it or not.

That force has a name. It's called "entropy."[1]

Entropy is one of the most well-established ideas in all of science. At its most basic level, it says this: without energy and maintenance being put in, everything naturally moves from a state of order to a state of disorder over time. Stars burn out. Mountains erode. Machines wear down. And bodies? Bodies are no different. The moment you stop actively working against entropy, it starts winning. Slowly, quietly, and without asking your permission, your body wears down. The Second Law of Thermodynamics, called "Entropy" states that everything is in a constant state of disrepair, meaning everything is in a constant state of returning to its original components. Human bodies are not immune from the same disrepair. But the corollary to the Law of Entropy is that it requires energy into the system to maintain it or improve it. That "energy," for example, is the new roof that your dilapidated house needs, and the glucosamine and Ligaplex and spinal manipulation that your degenerative disc disease at L3 to L5 needs.

Most people have never heard the word entropy used in the context of their own health. They think of it as something that happens to old bridges or abandoned houses. But the truth is, it is the single most important concept to understand if you want to make sense of why your body feels the way it does right now, and where it's headed if nothing changes.

Think about what happens to a car that sits in a driveway for three years without anyone driving it. The tires go flat. The battery dies. The engine seizes up. The rubber seals crack. The metal starts to rust. Nobody vandalized that car. Nobody did anything wrong. The owner just stopped putting energy and maintenance into it, and entropy did the rest. Your body works the same way. Stop maintaining it, stop moving it, stop giving it the care it needs, and the breakdown doesn't pause to wait for you to be ready. It just keeps going.

Now, here is what makes this personal. The breakdown does not happen all at once. You don't wake up one morning and suddenly find that your spine has collapsed or your nervous system has stopped working. Entropy is patient but constant. It chips away in tiny increments, day after day, year after year. A little stiffness in the morning. A little more tension in the neck by evening. A disc that's lost a fraction of its height compared to five years ago. None of it feels like a crisis. None of it sends you running to a doctor. But the process is absolutely real, and it's been underway for much longer than most people realize.

Your spine is one of the most complex and critical structures in your entire body. It's made up of 33 vertebrae stacked on top of each other, separated by intervertebral discs that act as shock absorbers or cushions, connected by ligaments and muscles that hold the whole thing together, and housing the spinal cord that carries signals between your brain and every single part of your body. That is an enormous amount of responsibility sitting in one structure. And like every other structure in the universe, it's subject to entropy. Without the right movement, the right care, and the right maintenance, it starts to break down. The discs start to thin out or wear out. The joints stiffen. The spaces where nerves travel start to narrow. And the signals that your nervous system depends on to run your body start to get disrupted.

That is not a scare tactic. That is anatomy. That is reality. And understanding it is the first step toward doing something about it.

Consider a hypothetical scenario. Picture a 44-year-old project manager named James. He sits at a desk for eight to nine hours a day, works out occasionally when life allows, and considers himself reasonably healthy. He doesn't have any serious medical conditions. He doesn't take any regular medication. He feels, by his own assessment, pretty okay. But over the last few years he has noticed that getting up from his desk takes a moment. His lower back feels tight after long drives. The more he sits, the more stiffness he feels when he stands. His right shoulder has started to bother him when he reaches overhead. He figures it is stress, or maybe he slept wrong, or maybe this is just what his mid-forties feel like. What James doesn't realize is that his spine has been quietly losing ground to entropy for years. The symptoms he's brushing off aren't random. They are the first visible signs of a process that started long before he ever noticed anything at all.

James's situation is not unusual. It is incredibly common. And it's exactly the kind of slow, quiet decline that this book is written to address.

Entropy does not discriminate. It works on athletes and couch potatoes alike. It works on people who eat well and people who do not. It works on twenty-year-olds and seventy-year-olds alike. The difference isn't whether entropy is happening to you. It's whether you are doing anything to push back against it. Because that is the only variable you actually can control.

The Decay You Can't Feel — Why Breakdown Starts Long Before the Pain

One of the most dangerous beliefs in health is this: "If I feel okay, I am okay."

It seems logical. Pain is your body's way of telling you something is wrong, so if there's no pain, there's no problem. The issue is that this belief is built on a misunderstanding of how pain actually works. Pain is not an early warning system. It's actually a late-stage signal. By the time your body is generating a pain signal strong enough for you to notice, the underlying problem has usually been building for months, sometimes years, sometimes decades.

Spinal degeneration is one of the clearest examples of this in all of medicine. Research consistently shows that significant structural changes in the spine, things like disc thinning, joint deterioration or degeneration, and narrowing of the spaces where nerves travel, can be present and progressing for years before a person feels any pain at all. Studies using imaging technology have found that a substantial percentage of adults with no back pain whatsoever show clear signs of spinal degeneration on their

X-rays and scans. The degeneration was there! The breakdown was happening. The person just could not feel it yet.

Think about that for a moment. Your spine could be losing structural integrity right now, and you would have no idea. Not because something is hidden from you, but because pain is simply not the tool your body uses to signal early-stage problems. Pain shows up late. It is the last resort, not the first notification.

A useful way to think about this is to compare it to tooth decay. A cavity doesn't hurt when it first starts forming. It is just a tiny area of breakdown on the surface of the tooth. You can't feel it. You can't see it without a dental mirror and a trained eye. But it's there, and it's growing. Weeks go by, months go by, and still no pain. Then one day, you bite into something and a sharp pain shoots through your jaw. By that point, the cavity has reached the nerve. The damage that took months to develop is now impossible to ignore. Your dentist doesn't say "well, this just happened." Your dentist says, "this has been building for a while." The spine works the same way. The pain you feel today is not the beginning of the story. It's usually somewhere near the end of tooth decay.

This is why the "wait until it hurts" approach to spinal health is NOT recommended and is so costly. Not just financially, though the cost of treating advanced degeneration is significant. But in terms of function, quality of life, and the options available to you. The earlier you address what is happening in your spine, the more you can do about it. The longer you wait, the more the breakdown compounds, and the harder it becomes to correct or reverse.

Your nervous system adds another layer to this. The spinal cord and the nerve roots that branch off it do not just carry pain signals. They carry every signal your brain sends to every part of your body. When aberrant spinal structures start to compress or irritate those nerve pathways, the effects are not always felt as pain. Sometimes they show up as fatigue.

Sometimes as reduced range of motion. Sometimes as digestive issues, headaches, poor sleep, or a vague sense that your body just isn't running the way it used to. These symptoms rarely get connected back to the spine because they don't feel like "back problems." But the spine and nervous system are at the root of far more of your daily health than most people ever realize.

The gap between how your body feels and how your body actually is can be enormous. Feeling okay is not the same as being okay. And once you understand that the whole idea of waiting for pain before taking action starts to look very different. You wouldn't wait for your brakes to completely fail before getting them checked. You wouldn't wait for a small leak in your roof to become a flood before calling someone. The same logic applies to your spine, and applying it early is one of the most powerful health decisions you can make.

You Are Either Moving Toward Health or Away From It — There Is No Standing Still

Your body does not have a pause button.

At every moment, at the cellular level, at the tissue level, at the structural level of your spine and joints, something is either being built up or broken down. Recovery is happening or deterioration is happening. There is no neutral state where everything just holds steady while you figure out what to do next. Biology does not work that way. Physics does not work that way. Entropy does not work that way.

This is one of the most important ideas in this entire book, so it's worth sitting with for a moment. Every single day, the choices you make are either slowing entropy down or speeding it up. How you sit at your desk. Whether you move your body. How you move your body. How much stress you carry and how your nervous system responds to it. Whether you get your spine checked and adjusted. Life is better adjusted! Whether you stretch, strengthen, and actively maintain the structures that keep you upright and functional. All of it matters. All of it is either adding to your account or withdrawing from it.

Most people think about health in terms of dramatic moments. The event. The injury. The diagnosis. The surgery. The recovery. But the reality is that health is built or destroyed in the small, quiet, daily moments that don't feel significant at all. The hours you spend hunched over your phone. The years you spend sitting in a chair that doesn't support your lower back. The workout you skip because you're tired. The stiffness you ignore because it's not bad enough to deal with yet. These things don't feel like decisions that matter. But they are. Every one of them is a vote, and the votes add up over time in one direction or the other.

Think of it like a bank account. Every good choice you make for your spine and nervous system is a deposit. Every bad habit, every ignored symptom, every day you spend in a posture that loads your spine incorrectly is a withdrawal. For a while, you can make more withdrawals than deposits and still feel fine, because you built up a reserve. But at some point, the account runs low. And when it does, the symptoms start showing up. The pain arrives. The stiffness becomes constant. The function starts to slip. And by that point, you're not just trying to get healthy. You are trying to climb out of a deficit that took years to build.

The good news is that this works in both directions. Just as consistent neglect compounds into breakdown, consistent care compounds into recovery and strength. Every good choice stacks on top of the last one. Every spinal adjustment, every intentional movement, every healthy habit that supports your spinal health is a deposit that builds on itself over time. You don't need to be perfect. You just need to be consistently moving in the right direction.

This concept gives you something that a lot of health conversations do not: real agency. You are not a passive victim of aging. You are not just watching helplessly as your body declines. You are an active participant in the direction your body is moving, and you have far more influence over that direction than you've probably been led to believe. The choices you make today matter. They matter tomorrow. They matter ten years from now. And the best time to start making better ones is always right now, regardless of where you are starting from!

Some people read this and feel motivated. Others feel a sting of guilt about the years they spent not knowing this. If you're in the second group, let that feeling go. You can't go back and change what you didn't know. But you can change what you do with what you know right now. That is where your power is!

The Good News — Entropy Can Be Slowed, Stopped, and Reversed

Everything you've read so far might sound like a long series of warnings. And in a sense, it is. But warnings only matter if there's something you can actually do about them. So, this is the part where the story changes.

Entropy is real. Spinal degeneration is real. The silent breakdown that happens long before pain shows up is real. All of that is true. But here's what's equally true: Your body has a remarkable, built-in capacity to heal, adapt, and recover when it's given the right conditions to do so. That capacity doesn't disappear when you hit forty, or fifty, or sixty or seventy. It is still there. The question is whether the conditions for healing are actually in place.

The human body is not a static structure. It is constantly remodeling itself. Your bones respond to load by getting stronger. Your discs respond to movement by staying hydrated and resilient. Your muscles adapt to the demands you place on them. Your nervous system rewires itself based on the signals it receives. This is called "neuroplasticity"[2] and structural adaptability, and it means that the breakdown you have experienced is not necessarily permanent. With the right input, your body can adapt and rebuild. It can restore function. It can reduce pain, improve mobility, and operate at a level you might have written off as impossible.

Spinal manipulation therapy is one of the most well-researched tools available for pushing back against the effects of entropy on the spine and nervous system. When a chiropractor performs a spinal adjustment, they are not just moving bones around. They are restoring proper motion to joints that have become restricted, reducing pressure on nerve pathways, and sending a powerful signal to the nervous system that changes the way the brain processes information from that area of the body. The research on this is solid. Studies show that spinal manipulation reduces pain, improves range of motion, decreases muscle tension, and has measurable effects on nervous system function.[3][4] It is not a fringe idea. It is a well-documented, clinically supported intervention that has been helping people recover function for many centuries.

But spinal manipulation goes beyond just pain relief, and this is the part that surprises most people. When the spine is properly aligned and moving the way it's designed to, the nervous system can do its job without interference. And when the nervous system is running without interference, the effects ripple out into every system and every cell in the body. Sleep improves. Energy levels go up. Immune function gets better. Digestion works more smoothly. Mood stabilizes. Focus sharpens. These are not coincidences or placebo effects. They are the predictable results of a nervous system that is finally able to communicate clearly with the body it controls.

Rehabilitation plays a critical role here as well. Spinal adjustments restore motion and reduce nerve interference, but building the muscular support around the spine is what makes those changes last. Targeted exercises that strengthen the deep stabilizing muscles of the core and back give the spine the structural support it needs to hold its alignment under the demands of daily life. Physical therapy approaches that focus on restoring movement patterns, correcting posture, and retraining the body to move efficiently work together with spinal care to create lasting results rather than just temporary relief.

The concept that ties all of this together is something chiropractors call Innate Intelligence. Your body already knows how to heal. It's been doing it your whole life. Every time you have recovered from an illness, healed a cut, or bounced back from an injury, that was your innate intelligence at work. The nervous system coordinates all of it. Innate Intelligence is the master controller, and the spine is the structure that either protects that controller or compromises it. When the spine is healthy and the nervous system is free from interference, your innate intelligence can do its job at full capacity. When the spine breaks down and nerve signals get disrupted, that healing capacity gets dialed back. Restoring spinal health isn't just about your back. It's about giving your body's built-in healing system the clear pathway it needs to function the way it was designed to.

None of this requires you to be starting from a perfect place. Whether you've been dealing with chronic pain for years, or you are just starting to notice the early signs of decline, or you feel pretty good and want to stay that way, the same principles apply. The body responds to good care at every age and every stage. People in their sixties and seventies who commit to spinal health and consistent movement routinely report improvements that they never expected. The research backs this up. It's not too late. It is genuinely never too late to start pushing back against entropy and giving your body the conditions it needs to rebuild.

Return to work. Return to play. Return to function. These aren't just clinical phrases. They're descriptions of what actually happens when people take their spinal health seriously and commit to a plan. The 55-year-old who gets back to hiking regularly. The office worker who sits through a full workday without pain for the first time in three years. The grandparent who can pick up their grandchildren without bracing for impact. These outcomes are real, they're achievable, and they are what this book is ultimately pointing toward. Not just surviving into old age but functioning well enough to actually live the life you want and thrive.

"A man is as old as his spinal column."

—Chinese Proverb

Putting It Into Practice

This chapter has covered a lot of ground, and it's worth taking a moment to turn the ideas into something concrete you can act on right now. Understanding entropy is valuable. Doing something about it is what actually changes things.

Start with this: Take two minutes and do a quiet, honest scan of your body. Not a dramatic inventory of everything that hurts, just a calm, clear-eyed look at what you notice. Is there stiffness somewhere that's been there for a while? A joint that doesn't move the way it used to? A recurring ache that you've been explaining away? Write it down. One area, one observation, one honest note to yourself. This is the starting point. You can't address what you haven't acknowledged.

Second, make one specific decision today about how you're going to sit, move, or carry yourself differently. If you sit at a desk, set a timer to stand up and move for two minutes every forty-five minutes. If you've been sleeping on a mattress that leaves you stiff every morning, commit to researching a replacement this week. If you haven't had your spine assessed by a chiropractor, book that appointment. Not someday. This week. One specific, scheduled action. That's what separates good intentions from actual change.

Third, shift the mental model you've been using to evaluate your health. Starting today, "I don't feel any pain" is no longer enough information. The new standard is: "Am I actively maintaining my spine and nervous system, or am I just waiting to see what breaks?" That shift in thinking is more powerful than any single exercise or treatment because it changes the decisions you make every day going forward.

Entropy is real. The breakdown is happening. But so is your ability to push back against it, and every good choice you make from this point forward is a step in the right direction.

A Brief History of Chiropractic — The Rebels Who Figured Out the Body's Master Switch

✦✦✦

Where It All Started — D.D. Palmer and the First Adjustment

In September of 1895, a self-taught healer in Davenport, Iowa made a decision that would eventually change the lives of hundreds of millions of people. His name was Daniel David Palmer, and he was about to do something that had never been done before in recorded medical history.

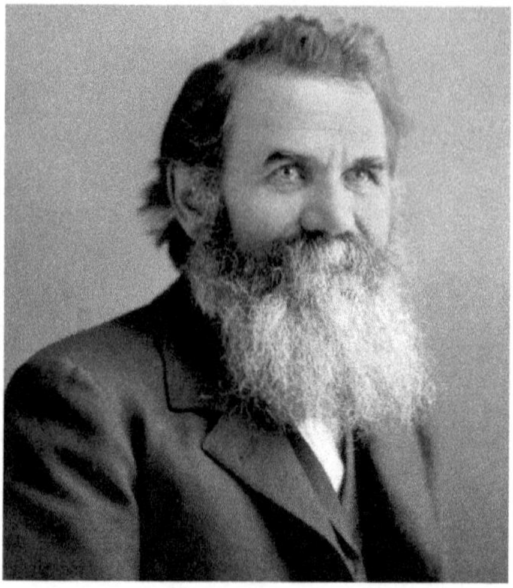

Daniel David (D.D.) Palmer
Discoverer of Chiropractic
Copyright: Public Domain Photo

The man on the receiving end was Harvey Lillard, a janitor who worked in the same building as Palmer's office. Mr. Lillard had been nearly deaf for seventeen years. He told Palmer that the hearing loss had started after he felt something "give way" in his back while he was working in a cramped, awkward position. Palmer examined Lillard's spine and found a vertebra in the upper back that felt noticeably out of its normal position. Using his hands, Palmer applied a specific, controlled thrust to that vertebra. Shortly after, Lillard reported that his hearing had returned.

One adjustment. Seventeen years of hearing loss. Gone.

Now, it's worth being clear about something. That single case didn't prove anything. One story does not build a science. And chiropractic has evolved enormously since that first adjustment in 1895. But what that moment did was open a door. It raised a question that medicine had not seriously asked yet: What if the spine, and the nervous system it houses, is connected to far more of the body's functions than anyone had previously considered?

D.D. Palmer wasn't a medical doctor. He was a self-educated man with a deep interest in human anatomy, magnetic healing, and the emerging understanding of the nervous system that was developing in the late 1800s. He read everything he could get his hands on. He studied anatomy. He observed patients. And he developed a theory that would become the philosophical backbone of chiropractic care: The nervous system controls the body, and misalignments of the vertebrae, which he called "subluxations," could interfere with that control and cause disease and dysfunction throughout the entire body.

He called the body's built-in ability to heal itself "Innate Intelligence." Ring a bell? Sound familiar? The idea was straightforward. Your body already knows how to run itself. It knows how to heal a cut, fight an infection, regulate your temperature, and coordinate thousands of simultaneous processes without you consciously thinking about any of it. The nervous system is the communication network that makes all of that possible. And the spine is the structure that either protects that network or compromises it. When a vertebra shifts out of its proper position and puts pressure on a nerve, the signal gets disrupted. The body's ability to self-regulate gets dialed back. Restore the alignment, restore the signal, and the body can do what it was designed to do.

That idea was radical in 1895. In many ways, it still challenges how conventional medicine thinks about the body today. But it was also, at its core, a deeply logical idea. And it was one that Palmer's son, Bartlett Joshua Palmer (B.J. Palmer), would spend the next several decades fighting to prove and spread to the world.

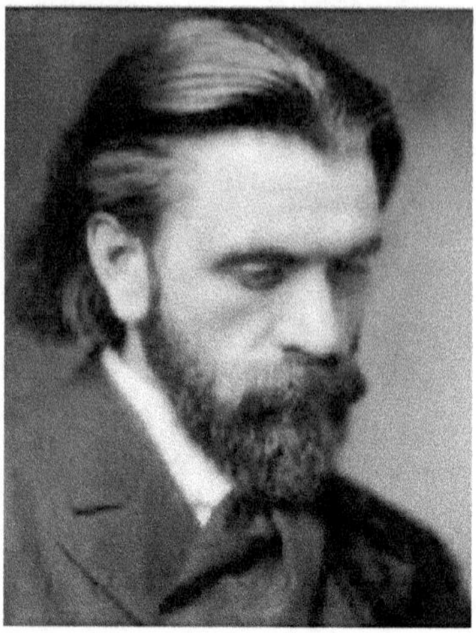

Bartlett Joshua (B.J.) Palmer
Developer of Chiropractic
Copyright: Public Domain Photo

B.J. Palmer took over the Palmer School of Chiropractic after his father and turned it into a powerhouse. He was a relentless promoter, a sharp thinker, and someone who understood that a good idea without a platform does not go very far. He built the school into one of the largest chiropractic institutions in the world, trained thousands of chiropractors, and pushed hard to get the profession recognized as a legitimate healthcare discipline. He invested in research at a time when almost nobody was funding it. He developed new techniques. He argued publicly, loudly, and persistently that chiropractic worked and that the medical establishment's resistance to it was more about politics and economics than it was about evidence.

He wasn't entirely wrong about that.

The early chiropractors faced serious opposition. They were practicing without medical licenses in a time when the medical establishment was actively working to define and control what counted as legitimate healthcare. Many early chiropractors were arrested and jailed for practicing medicine without a license. D.D. Palmer himself was jailed in 1906. These weren't people who were causing harm. They were people who were getting results, and the results threatened an establishment that had not produced those results itself.

That tension, between a new idea that was working and an institution that didn't want to accept it, would define the next century of chiropractic's development. And understanding it matters, because it explains why chiropractic still carries some skepticism in certain circles today, even though the science supporting it has grown dramatically stronger.

The story of chiropractic's birth is ultimately a story about curiosity. D.D. Palmer asked a question that most people were not asking. He looked at a man who had lost his hearing after something shifted in his spine, and instead of dismissing the connection, he followed it. He put his hands on a problem and tried something. That willingness to try, to question, to connect dots that the conventional thinking of the time said weren't connected, is exactly the spirit that eventually led to one of the most widely practiced healthcare disciplines on the planet.

Way Before D.D. and B.J. Palmer — Historical Evidence from the Georg Ebers and Edwin Smith Papyri

The ancient Egyptians developed one of the world's earliest systematic traditions of medicine. Two surviving texts—the Georg Ebers Papyrus and the Edwin Smith Papyrus—contain important observations about the musculoskeletal system, manual therapies, injuries, and the nervous system that bear interesting parallels to modern chiropractic concepts, although they do not necessarily describe chiropractic in the modern sense.

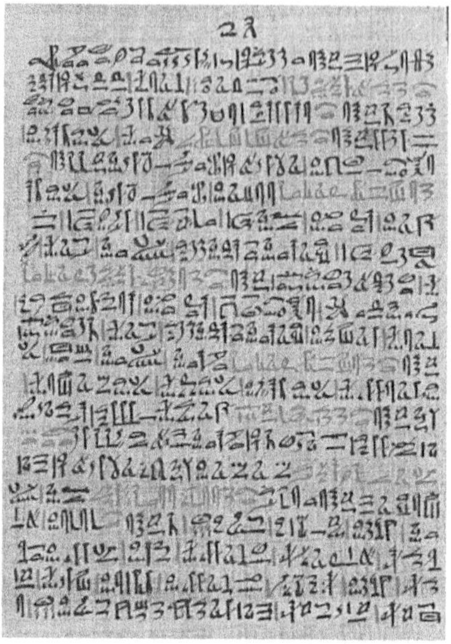

Georg Ebers Papyrus
c. 1550 BCE
Copyright: Public Domain

The Ebers Papyrus (c. 1550 BCE)[5], discovered at Luxor and purchased by German Egyptologist Georg Ebers in 1873, is among the oldest and most comprehensive medical documents ever found. It is believed to date back to 3500 BCE and contains more than 700 descriptions and discussions of anatomy, disease, and healing.

The Ebers Papyrus includes references to disorders and malpositions of bones and joints as well as treatments for muscular pain and stiffness including joint manipulation, massage, and manual rubbing of affected areas with or without various herbal concoctions. Ancient Egyptian healers recognized that injury and aging produced pain, swelling, deformity, and restricted movement. They employed combinations of heat, massage, and medicinal plants to restore function.

Although spinal manipulation or "chiropractic" is not explicitly defined or described, several themes of the Ebers Papyrus resonate with later chiropractic philosophy:

The importance of structural integrity to overall health.

The use of hands-on therapies to relieve pain and restore movement.

Recognition that disturbances in one part of the body can affect distant functions.

Emphasis on supporting the body's innate healing capacities.

These ideas represent broad healing concepts rather than direct antecedents of modern chiropractic adjustments. The Ebers Papyrus does not distinguish nerves from blood vessels as modern anatomy does. Instead, it describes a system of "metu"—channels or vessels—that extended throughout the body from the heart. The Egyptians believed these channels:

Connected all body parts.

Carried vital substances and forces.

Maintained bodily harmony.

Produced illness when obstructed.

While not equivalent to the nervous system, this concept reflects an early understanding that the body functions as an interconnected whole.

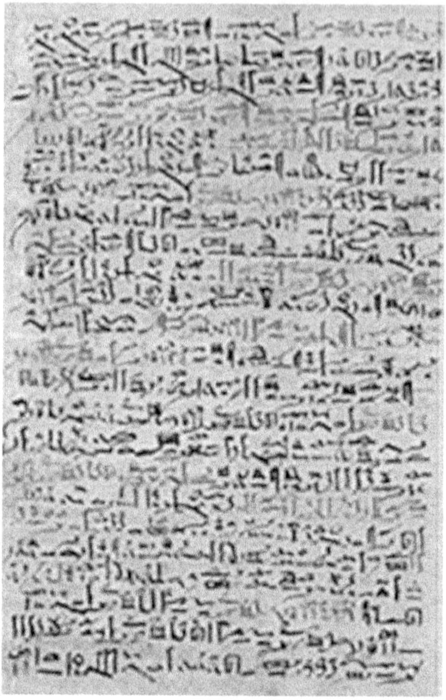

Edwin Smith Papyrus
c. 1600 BCE
Copyright: Public Domain

The Edwin Smith Papyrus (c. 1600 BCE)[6] is believed to date back to 3500 BCE (like the Ebers Papyrus) and is equally remarkable for its scientific and observational approach. Unlike the Ebers Papyrus, which includes manual therapies and magical remedies, the Edwin Smith text is primarily a surgical manual organized into 48 trauma cases. Many historians consider it the world's first treatise on surgery, orthopedics, and neurology. The Smith papyrus contains detailed descriptions of cervical spine dislocations, vertebral fractures, thoracic injuries, and lumbar trauma. Bone and joint alignment and stabilization were recognized as essential for healing. Manual repositioning methods are described for certain conditions, representing early forms of orthopedic and osteopathic manipulation.

The Edwin Smith Papyrus contains astonishingly advanced observations concerning the nervous system. The text includes the earliest known written reference of the brain. Egyptian physicians described cerebral convolutions, meninges, and cerebrospinal fluid. It also described the spinal cord and its apparent function in that injuries or disruptions to the spinal cord cause paralysis of the limbs, loss of sensation, urinary dysfunction, loss of speech, and loss of hearing.

Perhaps most significant from a chiropractic perspective is the explicit connection between structural injury or disruption and neurological consequence. Evidence from the papyrus shows that ancient Egyptian physicians understood that damage to the neck could impair movement and sensation throughout the body. This principle—that mechanical disruption of the spine influences bodily function—forms an important conceptual parallel to later manual healing traditions, even though the underlying theories differ substantially.

Neither the Ebers Papyrus nor the Smith Papyrus describes chiropractic adjustments, vertebral subluxations, or spinal manipulation as they are understood today. Nevertheless, both documents demonstrate that about 3,500 years ago Egyptian physicians appreciated several foundational concepts such as:

The body functions as an integrated whole.

Structural injuries and disruptions influence bodily performance.

Manual therapies can restore function.

Proper alignment of bones is important for healing.

The spinal column has profound effects on movement and function.

Careful examination and palpation are essential parts of treatment.

For these reasons, many chiropractic historians view ancient Egyptian medicine as part of the broader heritage of manual healing traditions that eventually contributed to the development of modern-day chiropractic.

What About That Hippocrates Guy?

Hippocrates of Kos, Greece (c. 460 – c. 370 BCE), also known as Hippocrates II, named after his grandfather Hippocrates I (also Hippocrates of Kos or Hippocrates I of Kos) was a Greek physician and philosopher of the classical period who is considered one of the most outstanding figures in the history of medicine and health. He is traditionally referred to as the "Father of Medicine" in recognition of his lasting contributions to the field, such as the use of clinical observation and prognosis, the systematic categorization of diseases, and the (later discredited) formulation of humoral theory. His studies set out the basic ideas of modern-day specialties, including surgery, urology, neurology, acute medicine and orthopedics, and advanced the systematic study of clinical medicine.

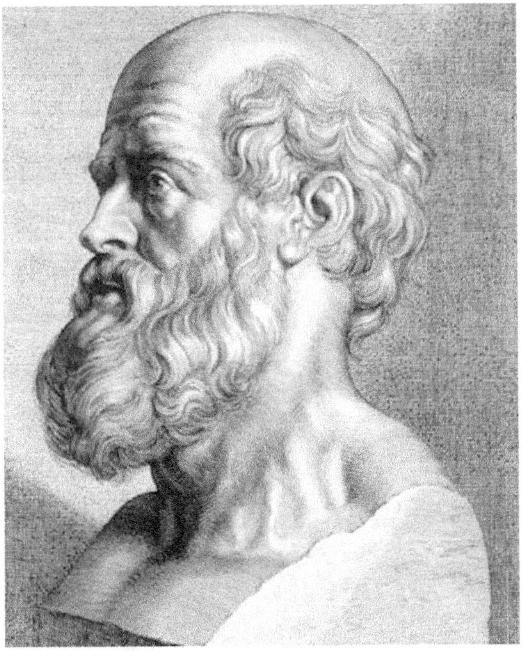

Hippocrates of Kos, Greece
Father of Medicine
c. 460 – c. 370 BCE
Copyright: Public Domain

Hippocrates is credited as the first person to believe that diseases were caused naturally, not because of superstition and gods. He separated the discipline of medicine from religion, believing and arguing that disease was not a punishment inflicted by the gods but rather the product of environmental factors, diet, and lifestyle habits.

"Look well to the spine for the cause of disease."
—Hippocrates

The famous advice to "look well to the spine for the cause of disease" is widely attributed to Hippocrates. It highlights the profound connection between spinal alignment, the nervous system, and overall health, serving as a core guiding principle in the field of chiropractic science and care. The philosophy behind this quote rests on the fact that your spine protects the spinal cord, which serves as the primary information highway between your brain and the rest of your body. When the vertebrae in your spine become misaligned—a condition sometimes referred to as a subluxation—it can create interference in the nerve signals transmitting from the brain to your organs and tissues. By correcting these misalignments through spinal adjustments, the nervous system can function optimally, allowing the body's natural healing processes to work without obstruction.

From Fringe to Mainstream — How Chiropractic Earned Its Place in Healthcare

For most of the twentieth century, chiropractic and conventional medicine were not on speaking terms.

The American Medical Association, or AMA, actively worked to discredit chiropractic care for decades. They labeled it an "unscientific cult." They discouraged medical doctors from referring patients to chiropractors or associating with them professionally. They ran campaigns designed to convince the public that chiropractic was dangerous, ineffective, and the work of charlatans, or worse, demons. This wasn't a quiet disagreement between colleagues. It was an organized effort to eliminate a competing profession.

The AMA's campaign was eventually brought into a courtroom. In 1976, a chiropractor named Chester Wilk, along with four colleagues, filed an antitrust lawsuit against the AMA and several other medical organizations.[7] They argued that the AMA had engaged in a systematic, illegal conspiracy to destroy the chiropractic profession. After years of legal proceedings, in 1987, a federal judge ruled in favor of the chiropractors. The AMA was found guilty of violating antitrust laws. The court found that the campaign against chiropractic had been carried out not because chiropractic was ineffective or dangerous, but because it was competition.

That ruling changed everything.

It didn't happen overnight, and the cultural shift took years to follow the legal one. But the Wilk case opened the door to a new era of chiropractic care, one where the profession could grow, research could be funded and published without systematic suppression, and medical doctors could refer patients to chiropractors without fear of professional consequences. The walls that had been deliberately built around chiropractic started to come down, and what was behind those walls turned out to be a substantial and growing body of evidence that the profession's critics had been working hard to keep out of public view.

The research that emerged over the following decades was compelling. Study after study showed that spinal manipulation was effective for back pain, neck pain, and headaches, often outperforming medication and other standard treatments while producing fewer side effects. A landmark report from the RAND Corporation in 1991[8] concluded that spinal manipulation was appropriate and recommended for certain types of back pain. The United Kingdom’s Medical Research Council published a study in 1990[9][10] showing that chiropractic treatment was more effective than hospital outpatient treatment for back pain. The evidence kept building, and it kept pointing in the same direction.

Think about a hypothetical scenario here. Imagine a 38-year-old physical therapist named Claire who trained in the 1990s and was taught, almost as a matter of professional culture, to be skeptical of chiropractic. Over the years, she kept seeing patients who had already been to a chiropractor before coming to her, and she kept noticing that many of them had already made significant progress. She started reading the research herself, not the opinion pieces, but the actual clinical studies. What she found did not match what she'd been taught. The evidence for spinal manipulation was solid, well-replicated, and growing. She started collaborating with a chiropractor in her area. Her patients got better faster. She never looked back. Claire's experience isn't unique. It's been repeated by thousands of healthcare professionals over the past three decades as the research has become harder and harder to dismiss.

Chiropractic's path into mainstream healthcare has been through several important doors. Sports medicine was one of the first. Professional sports teams began hiring chiropractors in the 1970s and 1980s, initially as an experiment and then as a standard part of their medical and training staff. The results were clear enough that the practice spread quickly. Today, every NFL team has at least one Doctor of Chiropractic on staff. So do NBA teams, MLB teams, and most Olympic national teams. Every NHL team employs a chiropractor. Every professional soccer team has a chiropractor on their team. The reason is not ideological. It is practical. Athletes who receive regular spinal care recover faster, perform better, and stay on the field longer.[11] When the goal is measurable performance, the evidence speaks for itself.

"Chiropractic just makes you feel so much better. When I walk out of the clinic, I feel like I'm about 3 inches taller, and everything's in place. As long as I see the chiropractor, I feel like I am one step ahead of the game."

—Tom Brady, Football quarterback

The military followed a similar path. The United States Department of Veterans Affairs began offering chiropractic care to veterans in the early 2000s.[12] The Department of Defense integrated chiropractic into military treatment facilities. The reasoning was straightforward: Musculoskeletal injuries are among the most common causes of disability in military personnel, and chiropractic care was producing better outcomes than many conventional approaches for those injuries. By 2019, there were active-duty chiropractors working in military treatment facilities across the country.

Hospitals began integrating chiropractic care into their multidisciplinary teams. Medical schools started including information about chiropractic and spinal manipulation in their curricula. Insurance companies, including Medicare and Medicaid in the United States, began covering chiropractic services. The profession that had once been jailed for practicing without a medical license was now licensed in all fifty U.S. states, regulated by professional boards, and practiced in some of the most prestigious healthcare institutions in the world.

None of this happened because someone decided to be generous to chiropractors. It happened because the evidence became too strong to ignore and the outcomes were too consistent to dismiss. The patients who were getting better made the case more powerfully than any argument could. When people who had been told there was nothing more that could be done for their back pain or neck pain walked out of a chiropractor's office with significantly less pain and significantly more function, that was the argument that ultimately won.

Chiropractic did not earn its place in mainstream healthcare by being loud or aggressive. It earned it by being effective, by building a research base, by training practitioners to rigorous standards, and by consistently producing outcomes that patients valued and that the data supported. The journey from a single adjustment in a Davenport office building to a globally practiced, hospital-integrated healthcare profession is one of the more remarkable stories in modern medicine. And it's a story that's still being written.

What Modern Chiropractic Actually Looks Like Today

Most people's mental image of a chiropractor is probably something like this: a back-cracking session in a small office, a few minutes on a table, some popping sounds, and you're done. That picture is outdated. And it's selling the profession dramatically short. It is quickly being referred to as rack 'n crack nonsense. And rightly so!

Modern chiropractic is a comprehensive healthcare discipline that addresses the relationship between the spine, the nervous system, and the body's overall function. Today's chiropractors complete four years of graduate-level education after their undergraduate degree, covering subjects including anatomy, physiology, neurology, radiology, orthopedics, nutrition, rehabilitation, and more. They are trained to read and interpret X-rays and MRIs, to perform detailed neurological and orthopedic assessments, and to develop individualized care plans that address not just symptoms but the underlying structural and functional causes of those symptoms.

The adjustment itself, which is the spinal manipulation that chiropractic is known for, is far more specific and sophisticated than most people realize. A chiropractor isn't just applying force to your back and hoping for the best. They are identifying specific vertebral segments that have lost their normal motion, applying a precise, controlled thrust to restore that motion, and doing so in a way that's calibrated to the individual patient's anatomy, age, and condition. The "crack" that people associate with chiropractic isn't bone grinding on bone. It is called cavitation, or more technically correct as tribonucleation. It is simply the release of gas from the fluid inside the joint, the same thing that happens when you crack your knuckles. The sound is a byproduct of the adjustment, not the goal of it. Not all adjustments result in cavitation or tribonucleation.

Beyond the adjustment, modern chiropractic practices often include soft tissue therapy, therapeutic exercise prescription, postural training, ergonomic counseling, and rehabilitation protocols designed to restore movement patterns and build the muscular support that keeps the spine stable. Many chiropractors work in integrated practices alongside medical doctors, physical therapists, massage therapists, and sports medicine specialists, sharing patient records, coordinating care plans, and communicating regularly about patient progress. The siloed, isolated practice model is giving way to collaborative care, and patients benefit enormously from that shift.

The range of people who see chiropractors today would probably surprise you.

Professional athletes use chiropractic care not just to recover from injuries but to optimize performance and function. A sprinter whose pelvis is even slightly misaligned is going to fire their muscles less efficiently, which means slower times and higher injury risk. A tennis player with restricted thoracic spine mobility is going to generate less rotational power in their serve. Restoring proper spinal mechanics doesn't just reduce pain. It directly improves how the body moves and performs, and at the elite level, that matters enormously.

Desk workers in their thirties and forties are one of the fastest-growing groups seeking chiropractic care. The modern work environment is extraordinarily hard on the spine. Hours of sitting in a forward-flexed posture, looking at screens at eye level or below, with shoulders rounded and the head pushed forward, loads the cervical spine at a rate that was never part of a healthy human design. The average human head weighs about ten to twelve pounds in a neutral position. For every inch the head moves forward from that neutral position, the effective load on the cervical spine roughly doubles. Someone sitting with their head four inches forward of neutral, which is extremely common in office workers, is putting the equivalent of nearly sixty pounds of load on their neck for hours at a time. Over months and years, that kind of chronic loading accelerates exactly the kind of spinal degeneration described in detail earlier and is discussed in even greater detail later in this book. Chiropractic care, combined with postural correction and targeted exercise, directly addresses this and corrects it.

Older adults are seeking chiropractic care more and more. The idea that chiropractic care isn't appropriate for people over sixty is a myth. Techniques are adapted for older patients, using gentler methods when needed, and the benefits are well documented. Improved mobility, reduced pain, better balance, and maintained independence are all outcomes that research has connected to regular chiropractic care in older populations. For someone in their sixties or seventies who is determined to stay active and avoid the slow slide into dependence that they watched their parents go through, chiropractic care is one of the most practical tools available.

Children and adolescents are also seen by chiropractors, particularly for issues related to posture, sports injuries, and the effects of heavy backpacks and prolonged screen use on developing spines. The spine is most adaptable during growth years, which means that addressing problems early, before they have decades to compound, produces some of the most significant long-term benefits of all.

The nervous system focus that D.D. Palmer identified in 1895 remains central to how modern chiropractic thinks about health. The spine is not just a structural column that holds you upright. It is the protective housing for the most important communication network in your body. Every signal your brain sends to your heart, your lungs, your digestive system, your immune cells, your muscles, etc., travels through or near the spinal column. When spinal structures are healthy and moving properly, that communication happens without interference. When they're not, the disruption affects far more than just your back.

This is why patients often report improvements in areas that seem completely unrelated to their spine after starting chiropractic care. Better sleep. Improved digestion. Fewer headaches. More energy. Reduced anxiety. These aren't mysterious or coincidental. They are the predictable result of a nervous system that's finally operating without the interference that had been quietly degrading its function. The spine is the gateway to the nervous system, and the nervous system is the gateway to everything else.

Return to work, return to play, and return to function are the goals that modern chiropractic measures itself against. Not just "your back feels better today." But: Can you do your job without pain? Can you play the sport you love? Can you pick up your kids and hug them, carry your groceries, sleep through the night, and move through your day with the kind of ease and energy that makes life feel worth living? Those are the real outcomes that matter, and they're the outcomes that a well-executed chiropractic care plan is designed to deliver.

The profession has come a long way from that first adjustment in 1895. It has survived legal attacks, cultural skepticism, and decades of organized opposition. It has built a research base that supports its core claims. It has trained hundreds of thousands of practitioners to high professional standards. And it has helped hundreds of millions of people recover function, reduce pain, and live better. That's not a fringe movement! That is a healthcare profession that earned its place the hard way, by working.

Your Next Move

Chiropractic was born from a radical but logical idea: the nervous system controls the body, and the spine is its gateway. Everything that's happened in the 131 years since that first adjustment in Davenport has either built on that idea, tested it, or confirmed it. The profession that once had its practitioners jailed is now integrated into hospitals, military facilities, and professional sports organizations around the world. That didn't happen by accident. It happened because the core idea was right, and the results kept proving it.

Understanding this history matters for one specific reason. It changes how you approach chiropractic care. When you know where it came from, why it was opposed, and how thoroughly it's been validated by research and real-world outcomes, you stop approaching it with vague suspicion and start approaching it with informed curiosity. And informed curiosity is exactly the right starting point for making a decision that could genuinely change and improve your health.

Here are three specific things to do right now, before you move on to the next chapter.

First, search for chiropractors in your area who specialize in spinal health and nervous system function. Don't just pick the first name that comes up. Look at their credentials, their approach to care, and whether they offer a comprehensive assessment that includes your full health history, spinal history, postural analysis, and a discussion of your functional goals, not just your pain symptoms. A good chiropractor wants to know where you want to get back to, not just where it hurts right now.

Second, book a consultation this week. Not a treatment session, a consultation. Most chiropractors offer an initial assessment where they can take X-rays if needed, evaluate your spinal alignment and range of motion, and give you a clear picture of what's actually happening in your spine. This gives you real information to work with instead of guessing. You can't make a good decision about your spinal health without knowing your starting point, and a proper assessment gives you exactly that.

Third, go into that consultation with specific questions. Ask about the state of your spinal alignment and spinal health. Ask whether there are any signs of early degeneration. Ask what a realistic care plan looks like for someone at your age and activity level, and what outcomes you can reasonably expect in thirty, sixty, and ninety days. Specific questions get specific answers, and specific answers give you the clarity you need to commit to a plan that actually moves the needle.

The history of chiropractic is ultimately a story about what happens when someone refuses to accept that the status quo is good enough. D.D. Palmer looked at a problem everyone else had written off and asked what was actually causing it. That question started something that has helped hundreds of millions of people. The same kind of question, asked about your own body and your own health, can do the same for you.

Innate Intelligence — Your Body Already Knows How to Heal Itself

✦✦✦

What Innate Intelligence Is and Why It Changes Everything

Right now, without any conscious effort from you, your body is doing thousands of things simultaneously. Your heart is beating at exactly the right rate for what you're doing at this moment. Your immune system is identifying and neutralizing threats you'll never know about. Your digestive system is breaking down your last meal and deciding what to absorb and what to discard. Your lungs are adjusting your breathing based on the oxygen demands of your tissues. If you have a small cut somewhere on your body, a precise, coordinated repair process involving multiple cell types and chemical signals is already underway. You didn't schedule any of that. You didn't think about it. You didn't have to.

That is Innate Intelligence at work.

The term was used by D.D. Palmer, the founder or discoverer of chiropractic, and while the word "intelligence" might make it sound abstract or philosophical, the concept itself is completely grounded in biology. Innate intelligence is simply your body's built-in capacity to self-regulate, self-heal, and self-organize. It is the operating system running underneath everything. The nervous system is how that intelligence communicates. And the spine is the structure that either protects that communication network or interferes with it.

Most people have never thought about their body this way. The typical model most of us grow up with is reactive. Something goes wrong, you go to a doctor, the doctor fixes it. The body is treated like a machine that breaks down and needs an external expert to repair it. That model is not entirely wrong, but it's radically incomplete. It completely leaves out the most important player in your health, which is your body itself. Your body isn't a passive object waiting to be fixed from the outside. It's an active, intelligent system that is constantly working to maintain order, repair damage, and keep you functioning at the highest level possible given the conditions it's operating in.

The conditions it's operating in. That phrase matters a lot!

Innate intelligence is always present. It never takes a day off. But its ability to actually do its job depends entirely on the conditions you create for it. Give it a clear, unobstructed nervous system and the resources it needs, and it performs at an extraordinary level. Put interference in the way, whether that's poor nutrition, chronic stress, lack of movement, or a spine that's misaligned and compressing nerve pathways, and that intelligence gets throttled. It is still there. It is still trying. But it can't fully express itself when the communication network it depends on is compromised.

This is the idea that changes everything for most people when they really grasp it. You are not broken. Your body hasn't turned against you.

The pain, the fatigue, the dysfunction you're experiencing isn't your body failing. It is your body working as hard as it can under conditions that are making its job harder than it should be. The goal isn't to override your body or mask what it's doing. The goal is to remove what's getting in the way and let it do what it already knows how to do.

Think about what happens when you get a cut on your finger. You don't have to tell your body what to do. Within seconds, clotting begins to stop the bleeding. Within hours, white blood cells and macrophages enter the area to begin the repair process. Within days, new tissue starts forming. Within weeks, the wound is closed and the skin is rebuilding. You didn't manage any of that. Your innate intelligence did. The same process, scaled up in complexity, is happening in your spine, your joints, your muscles, and your organs every single day. The question isn't whether your body can heal. It's whether you're giving it the conditions to do so effectively and optimally.

Understanding innate intelligence doesn't just change how you think about chiropractic care. It changes how you think about your own body. Instead of feeling like a victim of your symptoms, you start to see yourself as someone who has a powerful internal healing system that needs the right environment to operate at full capacity. That shift in perspective is genuinely motivating because it puts you back in the driver's seat. You are not waiting for something external to save you. You are working to clear the path so your body can heal and save itself.

What Gets in the Way — Interference, Subluxation, and the Blocked Signal

Innate intelligence is always working, but it can only do its job when the signals get through clearly. The nervous system is the highway those signals travel on, and the spine is the structure that either keeps that highway open or starts closing lanes.

When a vertebra shifts out of its normal position, even slightly, it can put pressure on the nerve roots that branch off the spinal cord at that level. Chiropractors call this a “subluxation.” The word itself comes from the Latin for "somewhat dislocated," or literally “below the light” which gives you a sense of the scale. We are not talking about a dramatic, visible displacement. We are talking about a subtle shift in position that's enough to alter how that joint moves and how the surrounding nerve tissue functions. Small cause, large effect.

A good way to picture it is a garden hose. When the hose is straight and unkinked, water flows through it at full pressure. Pinch it anywhere along its length and the water flow drops. The water source hasn't changed. The pressure at the tap is exactly the same. But the output at the other end is reduced because something is getting in the way. A subluxation works the same way. The brain is still generating signals. The nervous system is still trying to communicate. But when a vertebra is pressing on or impeding a nerve pathway, the signal that gets through is weaker, slower, or distorted. And the body part or organ at the other end of that pathway doesn't get the full, clear message it needs to function properly.

Subluxations don't always hurt. That's one of the most important things to understand about them. Just like spinal degeneration can progress silently for years before pain shows up, a subluxation can be present and affecting your nervous system function without producing any pain signal at all. You might have a vertebra in your mid-back that's been slightly restricted for years, quietly reducing the nerve flow to your digestive system or your immune organs, and you'd have no way of knowing from the outside. No pain. No obvious symptom. Just a nervous system that's running at less than full capacity, and a body that's working harder than it should have to in order to maintain its normal functions.

How do subluxations happen? The honest answer is that they're almost impossible to avoid entirely because they're caused by the ordinary stresses of daily life. There are three main categories. Physical stress is the most obvious: car accidents, falls, sports injuries, repetitive strain from work, poor posture held for hours at a time, or even the physical stress of being born. Emotional stress is less obvious but just as real. When you're under chronic emotional and psychological stress, your muscles tighten, your posture changes, and the mechanical load on your spine shifts in ways that can cause or worsen subluxations. Chemical stress, things like poor nutrition, dehydration, alcohol consumption, and environmental toxins, affects the health of the tissues that support and surround the spine, making subluxations more likely to develop and harder for the body to correct on its own.

The cumulative effect of these stressors over time is exactly what entropy looks like at the spinal level. Each one on its own might be manageable. But layer physical stress on top of emotional stress on top of chemical stress, day after day, year after year, without any regular maintenance or correction, and the subluxations compound. The restricted joints become more restricted. The nerve pathways get progressively more compressed and interrupted. The body's ability to self-regulate gets slowly, quietly dialed back. And eventually, the accumulated interference reaches a threshold where the symptoms become impossible to ignore.

Consider a hypothetical scenario. Picture a 41-year-old nurse named Sandra. She's on her feet for eight to ten hours a shift, frequently lifting and repositioning patients, often twisting under load in ways that her body wasn't designed to handle repeatedly. She also carries the emotional weight of her work home with her most nights. She has been managing a dull ache in her lower back for about three years by stretching in the morning and taking non-steroidal anti-inflammatory drugs (NSAIDs) on the bad days. What she doesn't know is that she likely has a subluxation of her lumbar spine that's been there for at least two of those years. The nerve roots at that lumbar level are likely partially compressed. Her left leg is slightly weaker than her right, though not enough for her to notice consciously. Her bladder function is slightly less regulated than it should be, something she's chalked up to stress and her age. The pain is real, but it's only one of several effects that the subluxation is producing. The other effects are flying under the radar entirely but accumulating. This is a hypothetical example, but it reflects a pattern that chiropractors see regularly in clinical practice.

The effects of subluxation extend well beyond the area of the spine where the misalignment exists. Because the nervous system is a connected network, interference at one point can affect function at multiple downstream locations. A subluxation in the cervical spine can affect nerve flow to the arms, the shoulders, and even the organs of the chest. A subluxation in the thoracic spine can affect the nerves that serve the heart, lungs, and digestive system. A subluxation in the lumbar spine can affect the legs, the bladder, and the reproductive organs. This is why people who start chiropractic care for back pain sometimes find that other health issues improve as well. The connection is not mysterious. It is neurological. Fix the interference, restore the signal, and the body parts that were being underserved by that pathway start functioning better.

Understanding subluxation changes the way you think about your symptoms. A headache isn't just a headache. Fatigue is not just fatigue. Digestive discomfort isn't just something you ate. These symptoms might be exactly what they appear to be on the surface. But they might also be downstream effects of a nervous system that's operating with interference it has never had cleared. The only way to know is to have your spine properly assessed by someone trained to find and correct subluxations. Not to assume everything is fine because nothing hurts badly enough yet.

Removing the Interference — How the Body Begins to Heal From the Inside Out

Most people receive healthcare that works from an "outside in" approach. A drug is introduced into the body to produce a specific chemical effect. A surgery removes or repairs a damaged structure. A cream is applied to a surface symptom. These approaches aren't without value, and there are absolutely situations where they are the right tool. But they share a common limitation. They're doing something to the body from the outside, and they're typically targeting the symptom rather than the underlying cause of that symptom.

"The doctor of the future will give no medicine, but will interest his patients in the care of the human frame, in diet, and in the cause and prevention of disease."

—Thomas Edison

Chiropractic "works" from the inside out.

The goal of a spinal adjustment isn't to add something to the body or to override what the body is doing. The goal is to remove the interference that is preventing the body from doing what it already knows how to do. When a chiropractor identifies a subluxated vertebra and applies a specific, controlled adjustment to restore its normal motion and position, they are not healing the body. They are clearing the path so the body can heal itself. That is a fundamentally different model, and it's a more powerful one in a lot of situations, because it works with the body's innate intelligence rather than around it.

When a subluxation is corrected, several things happen relatively quickly. The mechanical pressure on the nerve root is reduced, which means the signal traveling through that pathway becomes clearer and stronger. The surrounding muscles, which had been in a state of protective tension (hypertonicity) around the restricted joint, begin to relax. Blood flow to the area improves. The joint itself begins to move through its normal range of motion again, which is important because spinal discs do not have their own dedicated blood supply. They get their nutrients through movement, through the compression and decompression that happens when the joints move properly. A joint that is not moving is a disc that is not getting fed. Restore the movement, and the disc starts receiving the nutrition it needs to stay healthy and resilient.

The nervous system response to a good adjustment is immediate and measurable. Research using electroencephalography, which measures brain activity, has shown that spinal manipulation produces changes in cortical activity within seconds of the adjustment.[13] Studies measuring muscle activation patterns have shown that adjustments change how the brain coordinates movement.[14] Research on pain processing has shown that spinal manipulation affects the way the central nervous system processes and perceives pain signals.[15] These are not minor, local effects. They are whole-system responses that reflect the fact that the spine and the nervous system are in constant two-way communication, and that correcting a problem in the spine changes what the brain receives and how it responds.

The inside-out model also explains why chiropractic care often produces benefits that seem unrelated to the spine. When the nervous system is freed from interference, the organs and systems it serves start receiving clearer, more complete signals. The immune system, which is directly regulated by the nervous system, can mount more effective responses. The digestive system, which is heavily influenced by the vagus nerve running through the cervical spine, can function more efficiently. The cardiovascular system, the respiratory system, the endocrine system: all of them are downstream of the nervous system, and all of them benefit when the nervous system is running without interference.

"Nature needs no help, just no interference."

—B.J. Palmer

Rehabilitation is the partner that makes these changes last. An adjustment restores motion and reduces nerve interference, but the muscles and ligaments around the spine have often adapted to the restricted, misaligned position over months or years. They've shortened on one side, lengthened on the other, and developed movement patterns that reinforce the problem. Without targeted rehabilitation, the spine has a tendency to drift back toward the position it's been held in. Specific exercises that strengthen the deep stabilizing muscles of the spine, combined with postural retraining and movement pattern correction, give the adjusted spine the muscular support it needs to hold its corrected position under the demands of daily life. The adjustment opens the door. Rehabilitation keeps it open.

Physical therapy approaches work hand in hand with this process. Soft tissue work addresses the muscle tension and fascial restrictions that develop around subluxated areas. Stretching protocols restore flexibility to structures that have shortened. Strengthening programs build the endurance capacity of the muscles that support the spine through long workdays and demanding physical activities. When these approaches are combined with regular spinal adjustments and a clear understanding of the underlying cause of the problem, the results are consistently better than any single approach used alone.

The inside-out model does not mean that outside-in care is wrong. It means that for a large category of health problems, particularly those rooted in nervous system interference caused by spinal dysfunction, starting from the inside and removing the cause produces better, more lasting results than starting from the outside and managing the symptom. The two approaches can coexist. But understanding which one addresses the root and which one manages the surface changes how you think about where to start and what to expect.

Trusting the Process — Why Healing Takes Time and What to Expect

One of the most common reasons people do not get the full benefit of chiropractic care is simple. They stop too soon.

They come in with pain, they get a few adjustments, the pain improves, and they stop coming. The logic feels reasonable. The pain is gone, so the problem must be solved. But as you now understand, pain is a late-stage signal. If it took months or years of subluxation and nerve interference to produce that pain, then the disappearance of the pain after a few adjustments does not mean the underlying problem has been fully corrected. It means the nervous system has been relieved enough of its burden to stop sending the alarm signal. The structural correction, the restoration of proper joint mechanics, the rebuilding of the muscular support, the full rehabilitation of the nerve pathways: that work takes significantly longer.

Healing happens in phases, and understanding those phases makes it much easier to stay the course when progress feels slow.

The first phase is relief care. This is the early period of treatment where the primary goal is reducing pain and acute dysfunction enough for the patient to function more comfortably. For most people, this phase lasts anywhere from a few weeks to a couple of months, depending on how long the problem has been present and how significant the structural changes are. Adjustments during this phase are typically more frequent, often two times per week, because the spine needs consistent input to begin shifting out of the pattern it's been locked into. This is the phase most people experience, and unfortunately, it's often where they stop.

The second phase is corrective care. Once the acute symptoms have settled, the real work of structural correction begins. The goal here is to address the underlying subluxations more completely, restore proper joint mechanics throughout the spine, and begin building the muscular and neurological support that will make the corrections last. This phase is longer, often three to six months, and the adjustment frequency typically drops to once a week or so. Progress during this phase is less dramatic than the initial pain relief phase, which is why many people underestimate how important it is. The changes happening during corrective care are deeper and more lasting than anything that happened in the relief phase. Skipping it is like stopping a course of antibiotics as soon as you feel better. The symptom might be gone, but the underlying issue hasn't been fully resolved.

The third phase is wellness care. Once the spine has been corrected and the supporting structures have been strengthened and retrained, the goal shifts to maintenance and optimization. Entropy is always there and always working. The stresses of daily life are always loading the spine. Regular wellness adjustments, typically once or twice a month, keep the spine moving properly, catch new subluxations before they have time to compound, and keep the nervous system running at full capacity. This is the phase where people stop thinking of chiropractic as a treatment and start thinking of it as a health practice, the same way they think about exercise or dental care. You don't stop going to the gym because you're in shape. You keep going because that's what keeps you in shape. The same logic applies here.

The timeline of healing also depends on factors that vary from person to person. Age matters, because tissues that have been degenerating for longer take more time to respond and have a lower ceiling for recovery. The severity and duration of the subluxations matter. Lifestyle factors like diet, sleep, stress levels, and physical activity all influence how quickly the body can make and hold the changes that care is producing. Someone who gets adjusted twice a week but spends eight hours a day in a posture that recreates the problem is going to progress more slowly than someone who combines their adjustments with postural correction, targeted exercise, and attention to how they sit, stand, and move throughout the day. Chiropractic care works best when it is part of a broader commitment to spinal health, not a standalone intervention.

What should you actually expect to feel during the process? The honest answer is that it varies. Some people feel significant relief after their first adjustment. Others feel a temporary increase in soreness as tissues that have been restricted for a long time begin to move again. This is normal and typically resolves within twenty-four to forty-eight hours. Most people notice gradual, cumulative improvement over the first several weeks, with better days becoming more frequent and bad days becoming less severe. Between adjustments, paying attention to how your body feels gives you useful information. Where do you feel more mobile? Where is the tension returning? What activities seem to aggravate things and which ones help? These observations help your chiropractor refine your care plan and give you a much clearer sense of how your body is responding.

The most important thing you can do during the healing process is communicate clearly with your chiropractor and stay consistent with your appointments. Consistency is the variable that matters most. The spine responds to repetition. Each adjustment builds on the last one. Missing appointments doesn't just slow progress, it can allow the spine to drift back toward its previous pattern, which means the next appointment is partly catching up rather than moving forward. Treat your appointments the way you'd treat a commitment that genuinely matters because it does.

Key Takeaways

Your body has an extraordinary built-in capacity to heal, regulate, and restore itself. That capacity, what chiropractors call innate intelligence, is always active. But it depends completely on a nervous system that can communicate without interference. When the spine is misaligned and subluxations are present, that communication gets blocked, and the body's ability to function at its best gets quietly dialed back, often long before any pain shows up to alert you.

Chiropractic care removes that interference. The adjustment doesn't heal you from the outside. It clears the path so your body can heal itself from the inside. That's a different model than most people are used to, and it's a more powerful one for the kinds of problems that have their roots in nervous system interference and spinal dysfunction. Paired with rehabilitation, postural correction, and consistent lifestyle choices that support spinal health, the results compound over time in the same way that neglect compounds into breakdown.

Real healing takes time. The phases of care, relief, correction, and maintenance, each serve a specific purpose, and skipping any one of them leaves the job unfinished. The pain going away is not the finish line. It's the starting gun for the deeper work that makes the change last.

Here are four specific things to act on before you move into the next chapter.

First, ask your chiropractor to walk you through which phase of care you are currently in and what the specific goals of that phase are. If you don't have a chiropractor yet, this is the question to lead with when you book your first consultation. Understanding the phase you are in changes how you interpret your progress and keeps you from stopping too soon.

Second, start a simple log. After each adjustment, write down two things: how your body feels in the twenty-four hours following the appointment, and one observation about where you notice either improvement or returning tension. This takes just two minutes and gives you a clear picture of your body's response pattern over time. It also makes your appointments more productive because you are bringing real, specific information rather than a vague sense of how things have been going.

Third, identify one daily habit that is working against your spinal health and replace it with something specific. If you sit for hours without moving, set an alarm on your phone for every forty-five minutes and stand up for two minutes when it goes off. If you sleep on your stomach, which puts your cervical spine in prolonged rotation, commit to transitioning to a side-sleeping position with a pillow between your knees to keep your spine neutral. Pick one thing, make it concrete, and do it consistently for the next ten, twenty, or thirty days.

Fourth, stop using pain as your only measure of whether your care is working. Start asking better questions. Are you moving more freely? Is the tension returning more slowly between appointments? Are you sleeping better? Do you have more energy during the day? These are the signals your innate intelligence is using to communicate with you. Learning to read them gives you a far more accurate picture of your actual progress than pain alone ever could.

The Nervous System — The Master Controller That Runs Everything

✦✦✦

Your Nervous System Is Not Just About Feeling Pain — It Controls Everything

Most people think the nervous system is basically a pain detector. Something hurts, the nervous system reports it, you deal with it. That is the whole job, right? Not even close!

Your nervous system is running your entire body, right now, without you doing a single thing consciously. It is regulating your heart rate. It is managing your blood pressure. It is telling your stomach how much acid to produce and when to move food along. It is coordinating your immune cells, directing them toward threats, and pulling them back when the threat is gone. It is balancing your hormones, adjusting your body temperature, controlling your breathing depth and rate, and managing the electrical activity in your brain that determines whether you feel calm, anxious, focused, or foggy. Every single one of those processes is happening simultaneously, all the time, and your nervous system is orchestrating every bit of it.

That is not a small job. That is the most complex management operation in the known universe, and it's running inside you right now.

When people think about their health, they tend to think in systems. The cardiovascular system. The digestive system. The immune system. The endocrine system. These feel like separate departments, each doing their own thing. But that picture is misleading, because every one of those departments reports to the same headquarters. The nervous system doesn't just influence those systems. It runs them. It is the reason they function in a coordinated way rather than as a chaotic collection of independent parts. Without it, none of them work properly. With it running clearly and without interference, the whole body operates as the remarkably well-designed system that it actually is.

This is why protecting your nervous system isn't just one health priority among many. It's the priority that all the others depend on.

Consider a hypothetical scenario. Think about a 48-year-old marketing director named Paul. He manages a team of 38 employees, travels frequently, and has been dealing with a combination of symptoms for the past two years that no single specialist has been able to fully explain. His sleep is poor and disrupted. His digestion is unpredictable. He gets frequent headaches that his neurologist says are tension related. His energy crashes by early afternoon every day. His blood pressure has been creeping upward. Each specialist he has seen has looked at their piece of the puzzle and offered a solution for that piece. A sleep medication. A digestive enzyme. A blood pressure medication. A recommendation to reduce stress. Nobody has connected the dots. What Paul doesn't know is that a series of subluxations in his cervical and thoracic spine have been quietly reducing the quality of nerve signals flowing to several of the systems producing these symptoms. His problem isn't five separate problems. It is one problem showing up in five places. This is a hypothetical example, but it represents a pattern that's far more common than most people realize.

The nervous system is the missing piece in most health conversations. You can optimize your diet, your sleep, your exercise routine, and your stress management, and still be leaving a huge amount of your body's potential on the table if the nervous system that controls all of those systems isn't running clearly and optimally. Everything else you do for your health works better when the nervous system is functioning without interference. And the single most important structure for keeping that interference out of the picture is the spine.

The Spine Is the Nervous System's Highway — And It Needs to Stay Clear

Your spinal cord is roughly the diameter of your thumb. It runs from the base of your brain down through the center of your spine, protected by the 33 vertebrae stacked on top of each other that form the spinal column. At each level of the spine, nerve roots branch off the spinal cord and travel outward to specific parts of the body. The nerves leaving the cervical spine in your neck serve your arms, shoulders, and several of the organs in your chest and upper abdomen. The nerves leaving your thoracic spine in your mid-back serve your heart, lungs, liver, stomach, and kidneys. The nerves leaving your lumbar spine in your lower back serve your legs, your bladder, your bowels, and your reproductive organs. Every signal your brain sends to any of those structures travels through the spinal cord and out through those nerve roots. Every signal those structures send back to the brain travels the same route in reverse.

The spine is not just a structural column that holds you upright. It is a protective tunnel for the most important communication highway in your body. And like any tunnel, what matters most is that it stays clear.

When the vertebrae are properly aligned and moving the way they're designed to, the nerve roots that pass through the openings between them have plenty of space. The signals travel cleanly in both directions. The brain gets accurate, real-time information about what's happening throughout the body, and the body gets clear, precise instructions from the brain. The entire system runs the way it's supposed to.

When the vertebrae shift out of alignment, through the cumulative effects of poor posture, repetitive physical stress, injury, or simply the entropy that was described earlier, those openings narrow. The nerve roots get compromised or compressed. The signals that travel through them become weaker, slower, or distorted. And the body parts and organs at the other end of those pathways start operating with less than the full information they need. Not dramatically, at least not at first. Just a little. But a little, sustained over months and years, adds up to a lot.

Think of it like a dimmer switch rather than an on-off switch. A compressed nerve doesn't usually cut the signal off completely. It turns it down. And a body running on dimmed signals is a body that is working harder than it should have to, producing less than it's capable of, and wearing out faster than it would with a clear connection. That is entropy operating at the neurological level, and it is happening in the background of millions of people's lives right now without them knowing it.

The relationship between spinal alignment and nerve function is not theoretical. It is anatomical. It is real science! The spaces where nerve roots exit the spine are called intervertebral foramina or neuroforamina, and they are sized precisely for the nerves that pass through them when the vertebrae are in their correct position. When a vertebra rotates or shifts even a few millimeters from that position, the size of that opening changes. Research has shown that it takes very little pressure on a nerve root, as little as the weight of a dime, to reduce the electrical transmission through that nerve by as much as sixty percent. A dime's worth of pressure. Sixty percent reduction in nerve function. That is how sensitive this system is, and that's why even small misalignments matter far more than they might seem to on the surface.

Spinal degeneration compounds this problem significantly. As the discs between vertebrae thin out over time, the intervertebral foramina get smaller even without any specific misalignment. Bone spurs, which are the body's attempt to stabilize degenerating joints, can grow into those spaces and press directly on nerve roots. Ligaments that thicken in response to chronic instability can encroach on the spinal canal itself. All of these changes are the structural consequences of entropy working on the spine over time, and all of them reduce the quality of the nervous system's communication highway. Keeping the spine healthy and well-aligned isn't just about avoiding back pain. It's about keeping that highway clear so the master controller can do its job without interference.

How Nerve Interference Shows Up in Ways You Would Never Expect

If nerve interference always showed up as back pain, this would be a much simpler conversation. You would feel it, you would know where to look, and you would address it. But that's not how it works. Nerve interference is remarkably creative in how it shows up, and most of the time, the symptoms it produces don't get connected back to the spine at all.

Chronic fatigue is one of the most common. When the nervous system is operating under constant interference, it uses more energy to compensate. Think of it like a computer running multiple background programs that are consuming processing power without you knowing about it. The system slows down. Tasks that should be easy become harder. The battery drains faster. People dealing with nerve interference often describe a fatigue that sleep doesn't fully fix, a heaviness that's there even after a full night's rest. They've often been told their bloodwork is normal, their thyroid is fine, their iron levels are adequate. The problem isn't in the blood. It's in the signal quality.

Recurring headaches are another one. The upper cervical spine, specifically the top two vertebrae, has an extremely close anatomical relationship with the structures that regulate blood flow to the brain and the tension in the muscles and connective tissue at the base of the skull. Subluxations in this area are one of the most common and most consistently overlooked causes of chronic tension headaches and cervicogenic headaches. People spend years managing these headaches with over-the-counter medication without ever addressing the cervical spine dysfunction that's producing them.

Digestive issues are frequently connected to thoracic spine dysfunction. The vagus nerve, which is one of the most important nerves in the parasympathetic nervous system, travels through the neck and influences the function of virtually every organ in the chest and abdomen. Compression or irritation of the nerve pathways in the thoracic spine can affect gut motility, stomach acid production, and the regulation of the digestive process in ways that show up as bloating, constipation, reflux, or unpredictable bowel function. These symptoms almost never get traced back to the spine by the specialists who see them.

Weakened immunity is another effect that surprises people. The immune system is directly regulated by the nervous system. Research has shown that spinal manipulation produces measurable changes in immune markers, including increases in the activity of natural killer cells, which are a key part of the body's defense against viruses and abnormal cells.[16] When the nervous system is running under interference, immune regulation becomes less precise. People find themselves getting sick more often, recovering more slowly, and dealing with inflammatory responses that seem out of proportion to the trigger. The connection to the spine isn't the first place most people look, but the research increasingly suggests it should be.

Brain fog, poor concentration, and mood instability round out the picture. The brain depends on a constant stream of sensory input from the body to stay calibrated and alert. When spinal dysfunction reduces the quality of that input, the brain receives less of the stimulation it needs to maintain sharp, focused function. Studies measuring cognitive performance before and after spinal adjustments have found measurable improvements in reaction time, mental accuracy, and processing speed following treatment.[17] The spine is not just a structural support. It is an active contributor to brain function, and when it's not working properly, the brain feels it.

The reason all of this matters so much is that it completely changes the way you should think about your symptoms. A headache you've been managing with ibuprofen for three years might be a cervical spine problem. The fatigue you've attributed to stress and aging might be a nervous system running on compressed signals. The digestive issues you've been treating with antacids might have a thoracic component that nobody has ever evaluated. None of this means that every symptom is a spinal problem. But it does mean that the spine and nervous system deserve to be on the list of things you check, especially when other approaches haven't produced lasting answers.

The Brain-Body Loop — Why a Healthy Spine Means a Sharper, More Resilient You

The nervous system is a two-way street. Most people think about it as a one-way system, the brain sends signals down to the body, the body does what it's told. But that's only half the picture. For every signal the brain sends down to the body, the body sends a signal back up to the brain. This constant, bidirectional conversation is what allows the brain to stay calibrated, adaptive, and accurate in its control of the body's functions.

The technical term for the signals traveling from the body back to the brain is proprioception and sensory afference. These are the signals that tell the brain where your body is in space, how much load your joints are under, what the temperature of your skin is, how much tension is in your muscles, and thousands of other pieces of real-time information that the brain uses to make constant micro-adjustments to everything it's controlling. The brain does not work in isolation. It works in response to what the body is telling it. And the spine is the single richest source of sensory input to the brain in the entire body.

The joints of the spine are packed with mechanoreceptors, which are specialized sensory cells that fire signals to the brain with every movement the spine makes. When the spine is healthy and moving through its full range of motion, these mechanoreceptors generate a constant, rich stream of input that keeps the brain active, alert, and accurately informed about the body's state. When spinal joints become restricted and stop moving properly, that stream of input drops significantly. The brain receives less stimulation. Its calibration becomes less precise. Its ability to coordinate movement, regulate systems, and maintain sharp cognitive function all take a hit.

Research in neuroscience has consistently shown that movement, particularly complex, varied movement involving the spine, is one of the most powerful drivers of brain health.[18] The cerebellum, which is the part of the brain responsible for coordination, balance, and the fine-tuning of movement, receives a massive proportion of its input from the spine and the joints of the body. When that input is reduced by spinal dysfunction, cerebellar function declines, and the effects show up not just in movement quality but in cognitive function, emotional regulation, and the brain's overall ability to adapt and respond to challenges.

This connection between spinal health and brain function is one of the most exciting and least discussed areas in the research on chiropractic care. Studies using functional brain imaging have shown that spinal adjustments produce changes in prefrontal cortex activity, which is the area of the brain responsible for executive function, decision-making, and emotional regulation. A 2016 study published in the Journal of Neural Plasticity found that spinal manipulation changed the way the brain processed information from the body, with measurable effects on cortical activity that persisted beyond the immediate post-adjustment period.[19] These findings suggest that keeping the spine healthy and mobile isn't just good for your back. It's a direct investment in your brain's performance.

Think about what this means practically. A spine that moves well is a brain that gets better input. A brain that gets better input stays sharper, more adaptable, and more resilient under stress. The person who maintains their spinal health into their sixties and seventies isn't just avoiding back pain. They're actively maintaining the quality of the brain-body loop that keeps them cognitively sharp, emotionally stable, and physically capable. The spine and the brain are not separate concerns. They are part of the same system, and you cannot optimize one while neglecting the other.

The sympathetic and parasympathetic nervous systems play a critical role in this picture as well. The sympathetic nervous system is your fight-or-flight system. It's designed to mobilize your body's resources in response to a threat. Heart rate goes up. Blood pressure rises. Digestion slows down. Immune activity gets deprioritized. Muscles tense. Blood flow shifts toward the limbs and away from the organs. This is an extraordinary system when it's activated appropriately and then allowed to switch off. The problem is that chronic spinal dysfunction, combined with the chronic psychological stress that most people carry, keeps the sympathetic nervous system switched on far longer than it was designed to be. The body stays in a low-grade state of emergency, burning resources, wearing down tissues, and suppressing the very systems it needs for repair and recovery.

The parasympathetic nervous system is the counterbalance. This is the rest-and-digest system, the state where healing happens, where the immune system does its best work, where digestion is efficient, where the brain consolidates memory and clears metabolic waste during sleep, and where the body rebuilds what the day has broken down. The vagus nerve is the primary vehicle for parasympathetic activity, and it originates in the brainstem and travels through the cervical spine before branching out to the organs of the chest and abdomen. Cervical spine health directly influences vagal tone, which is the measure of how active and responsive the parasympathetic system is. A healthy cervical spine supports healthy vagal tone. A restricted, subluxated cervical spine can reduce it, keeping the body tilted toward sympathetic dominance and away from the recovery state it desperately needs.

Getting the nervous system out of chronic sympathetic overdrive and back into a healthy balance between sympathetic and parasympathetic activity is one of the most important things you can do for your overall health. Spinal care is one of the most direct and effective ways to do it.

What You Can Do Right Now to Support Your Nervous System

Understanding how the nervous system works and why the spine matters so much to its function is genuinely valuable. But knowledge without action doesn't change anything. So, this section is about turning what you've learned into specific, concrete steps you can take starting today.

The first thing to do is audit your posture at the three places where most people spend the majority of their day: their desk, their car, and their phone. These are the three environments that do the most cumulative damage to the spine and nervous system, and they are also the three environments where small corrections produce the biggest long-term benefits.

At your desk, your monitor should be at eye level, so your head isn't tilting down to look at it. Your ears should be directly over your shoulders, not pushed forward. Your lower back should have a gentle inward curve, supported either by the chair's lumbar support or by a small, rolled towel placed at the curve of your lower back. Your feet should be flat on the floor, not crossed or tucked under you. Sit in your current position right now and check each of these points. If more than two of them are off, your desk setup is actively loading your spine in a way that accelerates degeneration every hour you sit there.

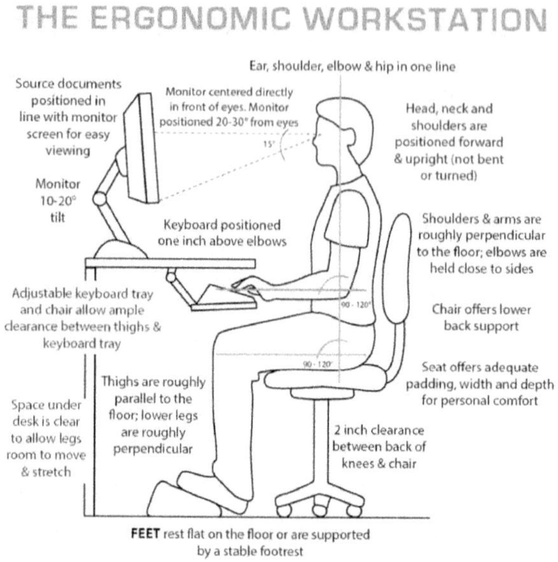

Copyright: Public Domain

In your car, the headrest should be positioned so the center of it contacts the back of your head, not the back of your neck. Your seat should be close enough to the pedals that your knee is slightly bent when your foot is fully depressing the clutch or brake, not stretched out straight. Your lower back should contact the seat back, not be hovering away from it. Long drives without lumbar support are one of the most common causes of disc compression and lower lumbar subluxation in working adults.

With your phone, the goal is simple. Bring the phone up to your eyes rather than dropping your eyes down to the phone. Every inch your head tilts forward to look at a screen adds significant load to your cervical spine, as described in detail earlier. If you use your phone for more than thirty minutes a day, which most people do by a significant margin, this single habit change reduces the cumulative load on your cervical spine more than almost anything else you could do without professional help.

The second action is to add one specific daily movement practice that targets spinal mobility. Not a general workout. Not a walk, though walking is excellent for other reasons. A targeted spinal mobility practice that takes less than ten minutes and directly addresses the joints that are most vulnerable to restriction from modern life. Here's a specific sequence you can start today.

Begin with ten slow chin tucks. Sit or stand tall, then gently draw your chin straight back, as if making a double chin, and hold for three seconds before releasing. This restores the natural curve of the cervical spine and activates the deep neck flexor muscles that support the head's weight properly. Follow this with ten thoracic extensions over a foam roller or a rolled towel placed across your mid-back, at the level of your shoulder blades. Lie back over it, support your head with your hands, and gently extend backward over the roller for three to five seconds at each level, moving the roller up your spine one vertebra at a time. This directly mobilizes the thoracic joints that become most restricted from desk posture. Finish with ten cat-cow yoga movements on your hands and knees, moving slowly and breathing into each position. Inhale as you drop your belly and lift your head, exhale as you round your back toward the ceiling. This mobilizes the entire lumbar spine and activates the deep stabilizing muscles that support it. Ten minutes. Every morning before you start your day. Consistency matters far more than the intensity.

The third action is to schedule a spinal assessment with a chiropractor who performs a thorough initial evaluation. Not just a quick look and an adjustment. Not that rack 'n crack nonsense! A proper assessment that includes orthopedic testing, neurological testing, postural analysis, range of motion testing, and spinal imaging (X-rays, etc.) if indicated. The goal of this assessment is to identify any areas of subluxation or restricted motion that may be producing nerve interference you're not feeling yet. Go in with specific questions. Ask which levels of your spine show restriction. Ask whether there are any signs of early degeneration. Ask what the nerve pathways affected by any subluxations are connected to in terms of organ and system function. The more specific the information you get, the better equipped you are to make decisions about your care.

The fourth action is to start supporting your parasympathetic nervous system deliberately, every single day. The most effective and accessible way to do this is through controlled breathing. Specifically, extend your exhale to be longer than your inhale. Inhale for four counts, exhale for six to eight counts. Do this for five minutes before bed. This breathing pattern directly activates the vagus nerve and shifts the nervous system from sympathetic dominance toward parasympathetic recovery. It costs nothing, requires no equipment, and produces measurable changes in heart rate variability, which is the most reliable measure of how well your nervous system is balancing its two branches. Combined with the spinal care that directly supports cervical vagal tone, this practice accelerates the shift toward the recovery state your body needs to heal and rebuild.

The fifth action is to start paying attention to symptoms you have been explaining away. Write down any recurring symptom that has not fully resolved despite your best efforts to address it. Fatigue that sleep doesn't fix. Headaches that come back regularly. Digestive issues that seem unrelated to what you eat. Mood instability that doesn't match your circumstances. Brain fog that comes and goes without obvious cause. These are not necessarily separate problems requiring separate solutions. They may be a single nervous system problem showing up in multiple places. Bringing this list to your spinal assessment gives your chiropractor the full picture they need to connect the dots between your spinal findings and the symptoms you have been living with.

Recap

Your nervous system controls every function in your body. Not most functions. Every function. The heart, the immune system, the digestive system, the endocrine system, the brain itself. All of it runs on signals that travel through the spinal cord and the nerve roots that branch off it at every level of the spine. The spine is not just a structural column. It is the protective housing for the master controller, and keeping it healthy, aligned, and mobile is the single most important thing you can do to keep that controller running at full power.

When the spine is compromised, the effects don't stay in the back. They travel along the nerve pathways to wherever those pathways lead. Fatigue, headaches, poor digestion, weakened immunity, brain fog, mood instability, and reduced cognitive performance can all be downstream effects of nerve interference caused by spinal dysfunction. Most people never make that connection because the symptoms don't feel like back problems. But the nervous system doesn't care what the symptom feels like. It only cares whether the signal is getting through clearly or not.

A healthy, mobile spine also keeps the brain-body loop running at full capacity. The rich sensory input that healthy spinal joints send to the brain keeps the brain sharp, well-calibrated, and resilient. The balance between sympathetic and parasympathetic activity that healthy cervical spine function supports keeps the body out of chronic stress mode and in the recovery state where healing, repair, and regeneration actually happen. These are not side benefits of spinal health. They are central outcomes of it.

Three things to act on before you move into the next chapter. First, do the posture audit today at your desk, in your car, and with your phone.

Identify the single biggest postural offender in your daily environment and make one specific correction to it before you go to sleep tonight. Second, start the ten-minute spinal mobility sequence described in this chapter tomorrow morning. Put it in your calendar as a recurring appointment. Treat it the same way you would treat a meeting you cannot move. Third, book your spinal assessment this week. Not next month. This week. You now understand enough about the nervous system and spinal function to know that waiting for pain before getting checked is the wrong strategy. The assessment gives you real information about what's actually happening in your spine right now, and real information is the only thing that leads to real decisions.

Fight or Flight Forever — How Chronic Stress Is Locking Your Body in Survival Mode

✦✦✦

The Two Modes of Your Nervous System — and Why Balance Is Everything

Your nervous system has two gears.

One is designed for emergencies. It's fast, powerful, and built to keep you alive when something threatens you. The other is designed for everything else. Recovery. Digestion. Immune defense. Deep sleep. Tissue repair. Growth. These two gears have names. The first is the sympathetic nervous system. The second is the parasympathetic nervous system. And the single most important thing you can understand about your health right now is that these two systems are not supposed to run at the same time. They are supposed to take turns.

The sympathetic system is your gas pedal. When it activates, your heart rate climbs, your blood pressure rises, your muscles tense, your pupils dilate, and blood flow shifts away from your organs and toward your limbs. Your body is preparing to fight or run. Digestion slows down because digesting lunch is not a priority when a threat is present. Your immune system gets temporarily suppressed because mounting an immune response requires resources your body is redirecting elsewhere. Your brain shifts into a narrow, threat-focused mode of processing. All of this is brilliant design. For short bursts, it's exactly what you need.

The parasympathetic system is your brake pedal. When it's active, your heart rate slows, your blood pressure drops, your muscles relax, and your body redirects its energy inward. Digestion resumes. Immune cells go back to work. Growth hormone gets released. Your brain shifts into a broader, more creative, more connected mode of processing. Your body starts repairing what the day broke down. This is the state where healing happens. Not kind of. Exclusively. Your body cannot fully repair itself while the sympathetic system is dominant. It's physiologically impossible, because the two systems are pulling resources in opposite directions.

The design was never meant to be a problem. For most of human history, the sympathetic response activated when a real threat appeared, lasted for a short burst of time, and then switched off. The threat passed, the parasympathetic system came back online, and the body repaired the damage. That cycle worked beautifully for hundreds of thousands of years.

The problem is what happens when the threat never fully goes away.

Modern life doesn't give most people clean, short bursts of stress followed by full recovery. It gives them a continuous, low-grade stream of stress that never fully resolves. The deadline that gets replaced by another deadline. The financial pressure that doesn't let up. The relationship tension that hums in the background. The phone that buzzes with demands at every hour. The body doesn't distinguish between a predator and a difficult email. It responds to perceived threat the same way regardless of the source. And when the perceived threat is constant, the sympathetic system stays on. Not at full blast, but at a low, persistent simmer that never fully switches off.

This is what scientists call sympathetic dominance, and it's one of the most widespread and least recognized health problems in the modern world. The body is stuck in survival mode, not because survival is actually at stake, but because the nervous system never gets a clear enough signal that the threat has passed. The brake pedal gets used less and less. The healing state becomes harder and harder to reach. And the body starts to pay the price in ways that seem completely unrelated to stress on the surface.

Sleep becomes fragmented because the sympathetic system keeps the brain in a state of low-level alertness that prevents the deep, restorative sleep stages from fully engaging. Digestion becomes sluggish or erratic because the gut is one of the first systems to get deprioritized when the body thinks it's in danger. Inflammation rises, because the immune system, which is supposed to be carefully regulated by the nervous system, starts operating without the precise parasympathetic oversight it needs to stay calibrated. Blood pressure stays elevated. Muscles stay tight. The body burns through its resources faster than it can replenish them. And slowly, quietly, the breakdown accelerates.

This is entropy operating through the nervous system. And it's happening to a very large number of people right now who have no idea that their chronic fatigue, their disrupted sleep, their persistent tension, and their slow physical decline are all connected to the same root cause.

The balance between these two systems isn't a luxury. It is a biological requirement. Without regular, genuine activation of the parasympathetic system, the body cannot maintain itself. It can't repair what breaks. It can't regulate what drifts. It can't fight what invades. The gas pedal was built to be used in short, powerful bursts. Keeping it pressed to the floor indefinitely doesn't just wear out the engine faster. It prevents the maintenance that would keep the engine running in the first place.

How Poor Spinal Health Keeps You Stuck in Fight-or-Flight

Most people understand that stress activates the sympathetic nervous system. What almost nobody knows is that poor spinal health does exactly the same thing, through a completely separate mechanism, running in the background twenty-four hours a day.

Your nervous system is constantly scanning your body for information. One of the most important categories of information it monitors is the mechanical state of your spine. The joints of the spine are loaded with sensory receptors that send a continuous stream of signals to the brain about position, movement, load, and tension. When those joints are moving freely and the spine is properly aligned, the signals they send are clean and reassuring. The brain registers normal mechanical function and maintains its baseline state without triggering any alarm response.

When spinal joints are restricted, misaligned, or under chronic mechanical stress, the signals change. The receptors in those joints start sending different information. Not necessarily pain signals, at least not at first. But altered mechanical signals that the brain interprets as a form of physical threat. The nervous system doesn't need to consciously identify the problem. It just responds to the signal. And the response to a signal that says "something is mechanically wrong here" is the same response it gives to any perceived threat. It activates the sympathetic system.

This means that a person with chronic spinal misalignment is walking around with their sympathetic nervous system being nudged toward activation by their own spine, all day, every day, completely separate from any psychological stress they're also carrying. The two inputs stack on top of each other. The emotional stress from work keeps the gas pedal partially pressed. The spinal dysfunction keeps it partially pressed from a different direction. Together, they push the nervous system into a level of sympathetic dominance that neither one alone would have produced.

Consider a hypothetical scenario. Think about a 39-year-old teacher named Rachel. She's been dealing with low-grade anxiety for about three years. She sleeps poorly, wakes up unrefreshed, and feels tense most of the day even when nothing particularly stressful is happening. Her doctor has suggested she consider medication for anxiety and has run bloodwork that came back normal. Rachel does yoga twice a week and tries to manage her stress, but nothing seems to fully take the edge off. What nobody has assessed is her spine. She has a history of a car accident six years ago that she considered minor at the time, and she's had persistent stiffness in her upper neck ever since. The subluxations in her cervical spine from that accident have never been addressed. They have been sending low-level mechanical stress signals to her brainstem for years, keeping her sympathetic nervous system in a state of low-grade activation that her yoga practice can partially offset but never fully overcome. Her anxiety isn't purely psychological. It has a physical driver that's been ignored entirely. This is a hypothetical example, but it reflects a pattern that research increasingly supports.

The anatomical reason this happens is specific. The upper cervical spine, particularly the top two vertebrae called the atlas (C1) and the axis (C2), has a uniquely close relationship with the brainstem. The brainstem is the control center for the autonomic nervous system, which is the system that governs the balance between sympathetic and parasympathetic activity. Mechanical dysfunction in the upper cervical spine directly influences brainstem function. Even subtle misalignments at this level can shift the autonomic balance toward sympathetic dominance in a way that no amount of breathing exercises or meditation can fully counteract, because the physical driver of the imbalance hasn't been removed.

The vagus nerve compounds this further. The "wandering" vagus nerve is the primary vehicle for parasympathetic activity, and it exits the brainstem and travels through the cervical spine before branching out to the organs of the chest and abdomen. Cervical spine dysfunction that reduces vagal tone doesn't just affect one organ. It reduces the overall parasympathetic activity across the entire body. Lower vagal tone means less rest-and-digest. Less rest-and-digest means the body spends more time in sympathetic dominance. More time in sympathetic dominance means less healing, more inflammation, worse sleep, poorer digestion, and a nervous system that's slowly burning out its own capacity to regulate itself.

Chronic spinal dysfunction also elevates inflammatory markers throughout the body. When the nervous system is in sustained sympathetic activation, it releases stress hormones including cortisol and adrenaline. Short-term, these hormones are useful. Long-term, elevated cortisol suppresses immune function, breaks down muscle tissue, disrupts blood sugar regulation, and accelerates the degeneration of spinal discs and joint cartilage. The stress that the spine is producing through nerve irritation triggers a hormonal response that then further damages the spine. It's a cycle that feeds itself, and it is one of the clearest examples of how entropy compounds when the underlying cause isn't addressed.

This is why addressing spinal health isn't just about managing pain or improving mobility. It's about removing a source of sympathetic activation that's keeping the entire body in a state of low-grade emergency. Every day that subluxations go uncorrected is another day that the nervous system is being pushed toward fight-or-flight by a physical input it can't override through willpower, stress management, or lifestyle choices alone.

The physical driver has to be addressed physically. That is what spinal adjustments do.

Turning On Your Healing System — The Power of the Parasympathetic State

Everything your body needs to repair itself happens in one specific state. Not during exercise. Not during your morning coffee. During parasympathetic activation. This is the state your body was designed to spend the majority of its time in, and for most people living in the modern world, it's the state they spend the least time in.

When the parasympathetic system is active, the body does things it simply cannot do while the sympathetic system is dominant. Growth hormone is released, which is the primary hormone responsible for tissue repair and muscle rebuilding. The immune system shifts into its most effective mode, with natural killer cells and anti-inflammatory cytokines operating at full capacity. The gut's enteric nervous system, which is sometimes called the second brain, coordinates efficient digestion and nutrient absorption. The brain clears metabolic waste through the glymphatic system, which is a process that only operates fully during deep sleep and deep relaxation. Inflammatory markers drop. Blood pressure normalizes.[20][21] Heart rate variability increases, which is the measure of how flexibly and efficiently the nervous system is regulating the heart, and one of the most reliable indicators of overall nervous system health.[22]

All of that stops, or significantly slows, the moment the sympathetic system takes over.

Spinal adjustments are one of the most direct and powerful tools available for shifting the nervous system out of sympathetic dominance and into parasympathetic recovery. The mechanism isn't mysterious. When a chiropractor corrects a subluxation, several things happen simultaneously that drive this shift. The mechanical stress signals from the restricted joint stop. The brainstem, which was receiving altered input from that area, gets cleaner information and recalibrates its autonomic output. The vagus nerve, if cervical spine function is restored, gets better support for its parasympathetic activity. And the mechanoreceptors in the now-mobile joint start sending the kind of rich, varied sensory input that the brain interprets as normal, safe, and non-threatening.

This is why people often feel a profound sense of relaxation immediately after an adjustment. Not just relief from pain, though that happens too. A whole-body release of tension that feels different from what stretching or massage produces. The muscles that were holding protective tension around the restricted joint let go. The nervous system shifts its output. Heart rate drops slightly. Breathing deepens. The body exhales, in a sense, at a neurological level. That experience isn't placebo. It is a measurable autonomic shift, and research using heart rate variability monitoring before and after adjustments has confirmed it consistently.

Research published in the Journal of Manipulative and Physiological Therapeutics found that spinal manipulation produced significant increases in heart rate variability following treatment, which is a direct measure of improved parasympathetic tone.[23] Other studies have shown reductions in salivary cortisol levels after adjustments, which indicates a measurable decrease in the body's stress hormone output.[24] These are objective, physiological changes that confirm what patients report subjectively: after an adjustment, the body feels different in a way that goes well beyond the local area that was treated.

Regular chiropractic care builds on this effect over time. A single adjustment produces a shift. Consistent adjustments over weeks and months produce a sustained change in the baseline autonomic balance. The nervous system spends more time in parasympathetic recovery mode. The cumulative healing that happens during that time adds up. Sleep quality improves. Energy levels stabilize. Inflammatory markers trend downward. The body starts to rebuild what chronic sympathetic dominance had been slowly eroding. This is the inside-out healing model that was previously described, operating at the level of the autonomic nervous system.

The combination of spinal care with intentional parasympathetic practices compounds the benefit significantly. Adjustments remove the physical driver of sympathetic activation. Specific daily habits then reinforce the parasympathetic state between appointments. Together, they create conditions where the body can actually do what it's always been trying to do: heal, repair, regulate, and rebuild. The next section covers exactly what those daily practices look like and how to use them in a specific, structured way.

Daily Habits That Shift Your Nervous System Toward Healing

Chiropractic adjustments do something that no daily habit can fully replicate. They correct the physical source of nerve interference that's driving sympathetic activation from the inside. But adjustments happen a few times a week at most. The other twenty-three or so hours of each day are shaped by what you do on your own. And what you do during those hours either supports the parasympathetic shift your adjustments are creating or works against it.

These aren't vague lifestyle suggestions. Each one targets a specific mechanism in the nervous system, and each one has a clear, measurable effect on the sympathetic-parasympathetic balance.

The most powerful daily practice for shifting the nervous system toward parasympathetic dominance is diaphragmatic breathing with an extended exhale. Here's exactly how to do it. Sit upright or lie on your back. Place one hand on your chest and one on your belly. Inhale slowly through your nose for four counts, directing the breath into your belly so that your lower hand rises while your upper hand stays relatively still. Then exhale through your mouth for six to eight counts, fully emptying your lungs before the next inhale. Do this for five minutes every morning before you check your phone, respond to messages, or engage with anything that requires a decision. The extended exhale is the critical element. It is what activates the vagus nerve and drives the parasympathetic response. Inhaling activates the sympathetic system slightly. Exhaling activates the parasympathetic system. Making the exhale longer than the inhale tips the balance in the direction you want. Five minutes of this practice every morning produces a measurable increase in heart rate variability that persists for hours after the practice ends.

Sleep is the most important parasympathetic state your body enters, and most people are doing several things that prevent them from getting into it fully. Two specific changes produce the biggest improvement for the most people. First, stop using screens with bright backlighting in the ninety minutes before bed. The blue light spectrum emitted by phones, tablets, and televisions suppresses melatonin production and keeps the brain in an alert, sympathetically activated state. This isn't a minor effect. Research shows that ninety minutes of bright screen exposure before bed can significantly reduce melatonin levels and delay sleep onset significantly.[25] Replace the screen time with something that doesn't require a bright light source. Reading a physical printed book, light conversation, or simply sitting quietly all work. Second, keep your bedroom cool. Core body temperature needs to drop slightly for deep sleep stages to engage. A room temperature between 65 and 68 degrees Fahrenheit (18 to 20 degrees Celsius) is the range where most people achieve their deepest, most restorative sleep. These two changes, combined, produce a more significant improvement in sleep quality than most supplements or medications.

Movement is essential, but the type of movement matters more than most people realize when it comes to nervous system regulation. High-intensity exercise activates the sympathetic system, which is appropriate in the right context and at the right time of day. But doing intense exercise within three hours of bedtime keeps the sympathetic system elevated during the hours when the body needs to be transitioning toward parasympathetic recovery. The most effective movement practice for nervous system regulation is low-to-moderate intensity, rhythmic movement done consistently. Walking is one of the best examples. A thirty-minute walk at a pace where you can hold a conversation activates the parasympathetic system, reduces cortisol, improves vagal tone, and produces measurable reductions in anxiety and sympathetic tone that persist for several hours. It also directly supports spinal health by loading the discs rhythmically through movement, which is how they receive their nutrition. Do this daily, not occasionally. The nervous system responds to consistent input, and one walk a week produces a fraction of the benefit of seven.

Social connection has a direct, measurable effect on parasympathetic tone that most people don't associate with nervous system health at all. The vagus nerve is activated by positive social interaction, eye contact, physical touch, and genuine laughter. Research by neuroscientist Stephen Porges, whose polyvagal theory has reshaped how scientists understand the autonomic nervous system, shows that safe social engagement is a powerful activator of the parasympathetic system available to humans.[26] This isn't soft advice. It is hard neuroscience. People who maintain close social connections consistently show higher vagal tone, lower inflammatory markers, and better autonomic regulation than people who are socially isolated. One specific action: schedule at least one face-to-face conversation per week with someone you feel genuinely comfortable with. Not a video call. In person. The nervous system responds to physical presence in ways that digital communication doesn't replicate.

Cold water exposure is a practice that surprises people with how quickly it produces a measurable autonomic effect. Ending your morning shower with thirty to sixty seconds of cold water activates the vagus nerve through a reflex called the diving response, which produces an immediate parasympathetic activation followed by a sustained increase in vagal tone that lasts for hours. The first few times you do this, the sympathetic system spikes first, which is the gasping and tension you feel when cold water hits your body. Push through that initial response and keep breathing slowly. Within about fifteen to twenty seconds, the parasympathetic system takes over. The research on cold water exposure and vagal tone is consistent and compelling, and the practice requires nothing more than turning the knob in your shower.

One thing that works against all of these practices is chronic phone use, particularly the habit of checking your phone within the first few minutes of waking up. The moment you engage with email, news, or social media, your brain is processing demands, evaluating threats, and making decisions. All of that is sympathetic activation. Starting your day with thirty minutes of sympathetic activation before your nervous system has had a chance to fully transition out of sleep mode sets the autonomic tone for the rest of the day in the wrong direction. The specific change is this: keep your phone out of your bedroom or put it on airplane mode overnight, and don't check it until you've completed your morning breathing practice and eaten something. This single habit change is one of the most consistently reported improvements in morning energy and overall stress levels among people who implement it, and the mechanism is straightforward. You're protecting the parasympathetic window that exists naturally in the morning and using it deliberately instead of immediately overriding it.

None of these practices are difficult. But they require consistency because the nervous system adapts to what it experiences repeatedly. One good night of sleep doesn't rebuild vagal tone. Thirty consecutive good nights start to. One walk doesn't change your autonomic baseline. Thirty walks in a row begin to shift it meaningfully. The same principle that makes entropy dangerous, the compounding of small inputs over time, is what makes these practices powerful when they're done consistently. Small, daily deposits into the parasympathetic account add up the same way small daily withdrawals do. The direction just changes.

Putting It Into Practice

Your nervous system was built to cycle between two states. One for responding to threats. One for healing from them. The problem isn't that the sympathetic system exists. The problem is that modern life, combined with the physical stress of spinal dysfunction, keeps it running far longer than it was ever designed to run. When that happens, the healing state gets crowded out, and the body starts breaking down faster than it can repair itself. That's not aging. That's a system that's been kept in the wrong gear for too long.

The good news is that this is one of the most reversible problems in the entire book. The nervous system is responsive. It changes based on what it receives. Give it the right inputs consistently, remove the physical sources of sympathetic activation through spinal care, and it will shift. The body will start spending more time in the state where it can actually heal. Sleep improves. Inflammation drops. Energy returns. The breakdown slows. That's not a promise of perfection. It's a description of what happens when a system that was running in emergency mode finally gets permission to stand down.

Here are three specific actions to take before you move on to the next chapter.

First, identify your top three daily stress triggers. Write them down on paper, not in your phone. Next to each one, write one specific, concrete change you can make to reduce that trigger's impact. Not eliminate it, just reduce it. If your biggest trigger is checking email first thing in the morning, the change is: no email until 8:30 a.m. If it's a commute that leaves you tense, the change is: play an audiobook or music instead of news radio during the drive. Specific triggers require specific responses. Vague awareness of stress doesn't change anything. A written, concrete plan does.

Second, start the five-minute diaphragmatic breathing practice tomorrow morning. Set an alarm for five minutes earlier than you currently wake up. Before you pick up your phone, before you get out of bed, do the breathing sequence described in this chapter. Four counts in through the nose, six to eight counts out through the mouth. Five minutes. Do it for seven consecutive days and pay attention to how your mornings feel compared to the week before. The difference is noticeable enough in seven days that most people don't need to be convinced to continue.

Third, bring a specific question to your next chiropractic appointment. Ask your chiropractor which areas of your spine are most likely contributing to sympathetic activation based on your current findings. Ask whether your upper cervical spine has been assessed, and if subluxations are present there, what the treatment plan is for addressing them. Ask how your adjustments are targeting nervous system regulation specifically, not just pain or mobility. These questions shift the conversation from symptom management to root cause correction, and they give you a much clearer picture of how your spinal care is working to restore the autonomic balance your body needs to heal.

Spinal Manipulation — What Actually Happens When You Get Adjusted

✦✦✦

It's Not Just 'Cracking Your Back' — Here's What's Really Going On

The sound stops people cold the first time they hear it.

A sharp, sudden pop. Sometimes a series of them. It comes from somewhere in the spine, and if you've never been adjusted before, it can feel startling. The natural assumption is that something dramatic just happened. A bone cracked. Something shifted violently. Something broke. None of that is true, and the gap between what people assume is happening and what's actually happening is one of the biggest barriers to people getting care that could genuinely change their health.

That sound has a name. It's called a cavitation, and it has nothing to do with bones cracking or anything breaking. Inside every spinal joint, there's a small amount of fluid that lubricates the joint and keeps it moving smoothly. That fluid contains dissolved gases, primarily carbon dioxide and nitrogen. When a chiropractor applies a specific, controlled force to a joint that has become restricted, the joint space opens slightly and rapidly. That rapid change in pressure causes the dissolved gases to form a bubble and release. The pop you hear is that bubble of gas escaping. It's the same basic phenomenon that happens when you crack your knuckles. No bones are harmed. No damage occurs. The joint is simply being moved through a range of motion it had stopped accessing on its own.

Not every adjustment produces a sound. Many techniques used by chiropractors are completely silent. The sound is a byproduct, not the goal. A chiropractor isn't aiming for a pop. They're aiming to restore normal motion to a joint that has become restricted, and the cavitation may or may not happen as part of that process. The quality of the adjustment has nothing to do with how loud the sound is or whether there's a sound at all.

What chiropractors are actually targeting is something called a fixation or a subluxation. As previous chapters have covered, a subluxation is a vertebra that has shifted slightly out of its normal position or lost its normal range of motion. It is not a dramatic dislocation. It is a subtle restriction that changes how the joint moves, how the surrounding muscles function, and most critically, how the nerve tissue passing through and around that area communicates with the rest of the body. The adjustment is a precise, controlled thrust applied to a specific vertebral segment at a specific angle and speed, designed to restore normal motion to that segment and reduce the mechanical stress on the surrounding nerve tissue.

The word "precise" matters here more than people realize. A chiropractic adjustment isn't a general shove to the back. A trained chiropractor spends years learning to identify exactly which vertebral segment is restricted, in which direction it has lost motion, and what angle, depth, and speed of force are appropriate to restore that motion for a specific person's anatomy and condition. The difference between an adjustment and someone pushing on your back is the difference between a surgeon making an incision and someone poking you with a stick. The external action might look similar to an untrained eye. The specificity, the intent, and the effect are completely different.

Think about a hypothetical scenario. Picture a 52-year-old contractor named Greg who has been waking up with a stiff lower back every morning for about four years. He's been stretching, taking ibuprofen on the bad days, and assuming it's just the toll of a physical career. He's never been to a chiropractor because he figures it's just "cracking your back" and he can do that himself by twisting in his chair. When he finally goes in for an assessment, the chiropractor identifies restricted motion at two specific levels of his lumbar spine and a rotational misalignment at his L4 vertebra. The adjustment applied to those segments takes about thirty seconds. Greg hears two pops. He gets off the table and notices that the deep ache he's had in his lower left side for years feels different. Not gone, but different. Lighter. The motion he'd been missing in that area starts to come back over the following days. Greg had been treating the symptom for four years without ever addressing the mechanical restriction that was producing it. This is a hypothetical example, but it reflects what chiropractors see in clinical practice every day.

How a chiropractic adjustment "works"

<u>For spinal levels C3 to S5:</u>

Adjustive force → Spindle fibers → Intermediolateral Nucleus of the Lateral Gray Column of the Spinal Cord (T1-L2) → Pontomedullary Reticular Formation of the Brain Stem → Fastigial Nucleus of the Cerebellum → Controls Tone

<u>For Spinal Levels C2 and C1:</u>

Adjustive Force → Spindle Fibers → Fastigial Nucleus of the Cerebellum → Controls Tone

The mechanics of what happens at the joint level during an adjustment are worth understanding in a bit more detail, because they explain why the effects go so far beyond just "loosening up" a tight area. When a vertebral segment becomes restricted, the surrounding muscles develop what's called protective guarding. They tighten around the restricted joint in an attempt to stabilize it, which makes sense as a short-term protective response. The problem is that this muscle guarding becomes chronic. The muscles stay tight long after the initial cause of the restriction has passed, and that sustained tension creates its own problems. It compresses the joint further. It alters movement patterns throughout the spine. It creates the kind of deep, persistent ache that most people describe as "muscle tension" but that doesn't fully respond to stretching or massage alone because the underlying joint restriction is still there driving the muscle response.

When the adjustment restores motion to the restricted joint, the mechanical input to the surrounding muscles changes immediately. The muscle spindles, which are the sensory organs inside the muscle fibers that monitor tension and length, receive a sudden burst of new information.

The protective guarding that was holding those muscles tight gets interrupted. The muscles can finally relax, not because someone stretched them from the outside, but because the mechanical reason they were contracting in the first place has been addressed. This is why people often notice that the muscles around an adjusted area feel softer and less tender immediately after the adjustment, even though no direct work was done to those muscles at all.

The joint itself also benefits directly from the restoration of motion. Spinal discs don't have their own blood supply. They get their nutrients through a process of compression and decompression that happens when the joint moves normally. A joint that isn't moving is a disc that isn't getting fed. Over time, the disc loses hydration, loses height, and becomes more vulnerable to damage under load. Every adjustment that restores motion to a restricted segment is also restoring the nutritional supply to the disc at that level. This is one of the reasons that consistent chiropractic care slows the progression of spinal degeneration. It keeps the discs moving, and discs that move stay healthier longer.

So, the next time someone describes a chiropractic adjustment as "just cracking your back," you'll know what's actually happening. A specific, targeted restoration of joint motion. A release of protective muscle guarding. A resumption of disc nutrition. And, as the next section explains, something far more significant happening in the nervous system at the same moment.

The Neurological Effect — Why an Adjustment Does So Much More Than Move a Bone

The mechanical changes that happen during an adjustment are real and important. But they're not the most significant thing that happens when a chiropractor performs a spinal manipulation. The most significant thing happens in the nervous system, and it happens faster than you can consciously register it.

The moment a specific, controlled force is applied to a restricted spinal joint, a massive burst of sensory input floods into the nervous system. The mechanoreceptors packed into the joint capsule, the surrounding ligaments, and the muscles fire simultaneously, sending a powerful wave of sensory signals up through the spinal cord and into the brain. This isn't a gentle trickle of information. It is a high-volume, high-speed burst of input that the brain hasn't been receiving from that area because the joint had stopped moving through its full range. The brain suddenly receives information it had been missing, and it responds immediately.

The first response is a rapid reduction in pain signals. The nervous system processes pain through a mechanism called the gate control theory of pain, which describes how non-painful sensory input can effectively close the gate on pain signals traveling to the brain. The flood of mechanoreceptor input generated by an adjustment competes with and overrides pain signals from the same area. This is why pain often reduces immediately after an adjustment, sometimes within seconds. The pain hasn't been blocked chemically. The nervous system has been given higher-priority sensory input that takes precedence over the pain signal. The gate closes. The pain signal gets turned down.

This effect is immediate, but it's also just the beginning of what the adjustment triggers neurologically. As mentioned earlier, research using electroencephalography, which measures electrical activity in the brain, has shown that spinal manipulation produces measurable changes in cortical processing within milliseconds of the adjustment. The prefrontal cortex, which is the area responsible for executive function, decision-making, and emotional regulation, shows increased activity following spinal adjustments. The motor cortex, which controls voluntary movement, recalibrates its output based on the new sensory information it's receiving from the adjusted area. The cerebellum, which coordinates balance and movement precision, gets a surge of input that improves its ability to fine-tune motor control. These aren't local effects confined to the area being adjusted. They are whole-brain responses to a change in the quality of information the spine is sending upward.

Muscle tone changes are another immediate neurological effect. When a spinal joint is restricted, the muscles surrounding it develop an abnormal tone pattern. Some become hypertonic, meaning they're chronically contracted and shortened. Others become inhibited, meaning they're under-active and not generating the force they should. This imbalance in muscle tone affects not just the area of the restriction but the entire movement chain above and below it. The body compensates. Other joints take on load that wasn't designed for them. Movement patterns become inefficient. Over time, these compensations create secondary problems in areas that seem unrelated to the original restriction.

The adjustment interrupts this pattern at the neurological level. The burst of sensory input from the corrected joint resets the motor output from the brain to the muscles in that area. Hypertonic muscles receive a signal that allows them to reduce their contraction. Inhibited muscles receive a signal that wakes them back up. The muscle tone pattern around the spine begins to normalize. This is why people often notice improved posture, easier movement, and reduced tension in areas they didn't even know were compensating, all from an adjustment to a specific segment. The nervous system doesn't think in isolated segments. It thinks in whole-body movement patterns, and correcting one piece of the pattern resets the whole thing.

HOW A CHIROPRACTIC ADJUSTMENT WORKS

A chiropractic adjustment produces a mechanical stimulus that is detected by spinal receptors. This information travels through specific neural pathways that influence the cerebellum, which plays a key role in controlling muscle tone.

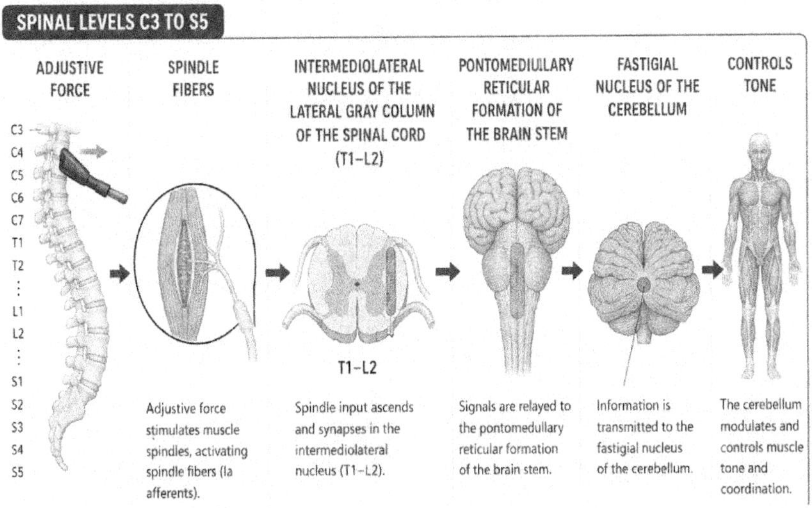

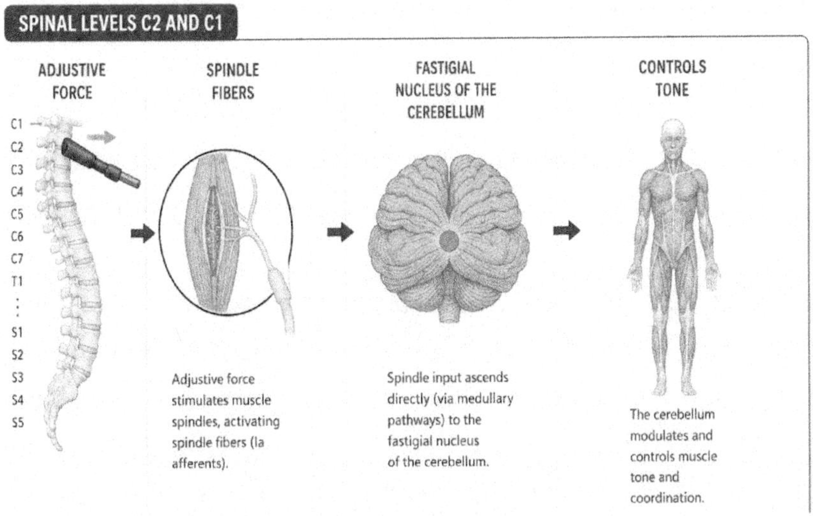

The neurological effects extend well beyond the musculoskeletal system. As previously described and explained in detail, the autonomic nervous system, which governs the balance between sympathetic and parasympathetic activity, is directly influenced by spinal mechanics. An adjustment that restores normal motion to a restricted segment also restores normal sensory input to the brainstem, which is the control center for autonomic regulation. The brainstem recalibrates. The sympathetic activation that the restricted joint had been driving through altered mechanical signals gets reduced. Parasympathetic tone increases. The body shifts toward the healing state. This is why people often report feeling calm, clear, and unusually relaxed after an adjustment. Not just less sore in their back. Genuinely lighter, clearer, and more settled throughout their entire body.

Research has confirmed this autonomic shift with objective measurements. As described earlier, studies measuring heart rate variability, which is the most reliable non-invasive indicator of autonomic nervous system balance, have consistently shown increases in parasympathetic tone following spinal adjustments. Studies measuring cortisol levels, which is the body's primary stress hormone, have shown measurable reductions following manipulation. And research on immune markers has found increases in natural killer cell activity following adjustments. These are not placebo responses. They are measurable, physiological changes in systems that have no reason to change unless the nervous system that controls them has actually changed its output.

There's also a phenomenon called proprioceptive recalibration that happens after an adjustment, and it's one of the most practically important neurological effects for people who want to move better and perform better. Proprioception is the sense of where your body is in space. It's what allows you to walk without looking at your feet, to reach for a glass without knocking it over, to catch yourself when you stumble. It depends entirely on accurate, real-time sensory input from your joints, muscles, and connective tissue. When spinal joints are restricted and not moving through their full range, the proprioceptive signals they send to the brain become inaccurate. The brain's map of where the body is in space becomes slightly distorted. Movement becomes less efficient. Balance becomes slightly less precise. The risk of injury goes up because the brain is working with a map that doesn't fully match reality.

An adjustment restores accurate proprioceptive input from the corrected joint. The brain's map updates. Movement efficiency improves. Balance improves. Reaction time improves. This is why athletes who receive regular chiropractic care consistently report improvements in coordination, agility, and precision that go beyond what their training alone produces. The spine isn't just a structural support for athletic movement. It is a major sensory organ that feeds the brain the information it needs to coordinate that movement accurately. Keep the spine moving properly, and the brain gets better information. Better information produces better movement.

The neurological effects of an adjustment also accumulate over time in ways that a single treatment can't fully capture. Each adjustment builds on the previous one. The nervous system learns from repeated, consistent input. As the spine receives regular corrections and begins to spend more time in proper alignment and full range of motion, the quality of sensory input it sends to the brain improves progressively. The brain's motor output becomes more accurate. The autonomic balance tilts further toward parasympathetic recovery. Pain processing becomes more efficient. The entire system runs better, not just on the day of the adjustment, but as a sustained baseline that improves with consistent care. This is the compounding effect of chiropractic care, and it's why people who commit to regular adjustments over months and years report improvements that far exceed what they experienced in the early weeks of treatment.

Is It Safe? Addressing the Concerns Honestly and Directly

Safety is the question that deserves a straight answer. No deflection, no overselling, no minimizing. Just honest information.

Spinal manipulation performed by a licensed chiropractor is one of the safest interventions available in musculoskeletal healthcare. The research on this is clear and consistent. Multiple large-scale reviews of the evidence have concluded that the risk of serious adverse events from chiropractic spinal manipulation is extremely low. A frequently cited systematic review found the risk of serious complications from lumbar spinal manipulation to be approximately one in several million treatments.[27] For cervical spine manipulation, estimates vary across studies, but the consistently reported range for serious adverse events is between one in 400,000 and one in several million adjustments, depending on the population studied and the definition of "serious adverse event" used.[28]

To put those numbers in context, consider what people routinely accept as normal healthcare risk. Non-steroidal anti-inflammatory drugs like ibuprofen and naproxen, which millions of people take daily for back and neck pain, are associated with approximately 16,000 deaths per year in the United States from gastrointestinal complications alone. The risk of serious complications from spinal surgery is orders of magnitude higher than the risk from spinal manipulation. Even acetaminophen, which is considered one of the safest over-the-counter pain medications, causes thousands of hospitalizations and hundreds of deaths annually from liver toxicity. Comparing the risk profile of chiropractic care to these alternatives puts the numbers in proper perspective. The option that gets labeled as risky is statistically far safer than the options most people use without a second thought.

The most commonly discussed risk associated with cervical spine manipulation is vertebral artery dissection, which is a tear in the inner lining of the vertebral artery that can, in rare cases, lead to stroke. This is the concern that gets the most attention in discussions about chiropractic safety, and it deserves a clear, honest response. The evidence on this topic has been examined extensively, and the current scientific consensus is that the association between cervical manipulation and vertebral artery dissection is far less clear than early reports suggested. A large population-based study published in Spine in 2008 found that the risk of vertebral artery dissection was no higher in people who had visited a chiropractor than in people who had visited a primary care physician for the same complaint.[29] The more likely explanation, supported by multiple studies, is that people who are in the early stages of a vertebral artery dissection often experience neck pain and headache as their first symptoms, which leads them to seek care from a chiropractor or a doctor, and the dissection completes on its own regardless of what treatment is given. The visit to the chiropractor doesn't cause the event. The event was already in progress when the person sought care.

This doesn't mean the risk is zero. No healthcare intervention carries zero risk. But it does mean that the risk of cervical manipulation has been significantly overstated in some media and medical circles, and that the actual evidence-based risk, when placed alongside the risks of the alternatives, supports chiropractic care as a genuinely safe option for the vast majority of people.

The most common side effects of spinal manipulation are mild and temporary. Studies consistently report that the most frequent post-adjustment experiences are mild soreness or aching in the treated area, similar to what you'd feel after a new exercise, and occasional temporary fatigue.[30] These effects typically resolve within twenty-four to forty-eight hours and are reported by roughly a third to half of patients at some point during their care. They are not a sign that something went wrong. They are a sign that tissues that have been restricted for a long time are beginning to move again, and the body is adapting to that change.

Chiropractors are trained to identify contraindications to spinal manipulation, which are conditions where manipulation is not appropriate or requires significant modification. These include active fractures, severe osteoporosis, certain vascular conditions, active infections in the spinal area, and specific neurological emergencies. A thorough initial assessment, which includes a detailed health history, physical examination, and imaging when indicated, is specifically designed to identify these contraindications before any treatment begins. A competent chiropractor will refer out or modify their approach when contraindications are present. The assessment isn't a formality. It's a critical safety step that shapes the entire care plan.

People with osteoporosis, a history of spinal surgery, or significant spinal degeneration are not automatically excluded from chiropractic care. They require a modified approach, using gentler, lower-force techniques that are specifically designed for more vulnerable spinal structures. Many chiropractors specialize in these populations and use techniques like flexion-distraction, Activator methods, or drop-table adjusting that deliver the neurological benefits of spinal manipulation with significantly reduced mechanical force. The idea that chiropractic care is only for young, healthy spines is a myth. The techniques available today are adaptable to a very wide range of ages, conditions, and structural situations.

The question of whether chiropractic care is safe is ultimately a question that deserves to be answered with evidence rather than with either blanket reassurance or exaggerated fear. The evidence says this: when performed by a licensed, properly trained chiropractor following a thorough assessment, spinal manipulation is a safe, well-tolerated, and effective intervention for a wide range of musculoskeletal and neurological complaints, with a risk profile that compares favorably to most of the alternatives people use without giving safety a second thought. That's not marketing language. That's what the research consistently shows.

One more thing worth saying clearly. Fear of chiropractic care, when it's based on misunderstanding rather than evidence, has a real cost. People who avoid getting adjusted because they've heard something scary and never looked into it further are people who continue living with pain, dysfunction, and nervous system interference that could be addressed. The cost of unnecessary fear isn't zero. It is the continued breakdown that happens while a person waits for a reason to act that never comes. Getting accurate information and making a decision based on that information is always better than making a decision based on something you heard and never questioned.

Your Next Move

A chiropractic adjustment is not a party trick, a placebo, or a rough shove to the back. It is a precise, targeted intervention that restores motion to restricted spinal joints, floods the nervous system with sensory input it had been missing, resets muscle tone, reduces pain signals, recalibrates proprioception, and shifts the autonomic nervous system toward the parasympathetic healing state. The effects are immediate and measurable at the neurological level, and they compound over time with consistent care into improvements that touch every system in the body. The safety profile, when examined honestly against the evidence, is excellent and compares favorably to interventions most people accept without question.

Understanding what an adjustment actually does changes how you approach it. You are not going in to get cracked. You are going in to restore the quality of communication between your spine and your nervous system, and to give your body's built-in healing capacity the clear pathway it needs to do its job.

Here are three specific actions to take before you move into the next chapter.

If you've been hesitant about getting adjusted, book a consultation this week. Not a treatment session yet, a consultation. Go in and ask every question you have. Ask the chiropractor to explain exactly what they found in your assessment, which spinal levels are restricted, and what their adjustment approach involves. Ask about any specific concerns you have based on your health history. A good chiropractor welcomes these questions because an informed patient who understands what's happening and why makes better decisions about their care and gets better results from it. The consultation costs you nothing but an hour of your time, and it replaces vague concern with actual information.

After your next adjustment, pay deliberate attention to how your whole body feels over the following twenty-four hours, not just the area that was treated. Notice your energy level. Notice whether your sleep that night is different. Notice whether areas of tension that you've stopped consciously registering feel any different. Notice whether your thinking feels clearer or your mood feels more settled. Write these observations down. Most people are surprised by how much they notice when they're actually looking for it, and those observations give your chiropractor valuable information about how your nervous system is responding to care.

Share what you've learned in this chapter with one person in your life who could benefit. Not as a sales pitch, just as information. The person who's been managing chronic neck pain with ibuprofen for two years. The family member who's been told their back pain is "just aging." The friend who's been avoiding chiropractic because they heard something scary about it once and never looked into it further. You now understand what actually happens during an adjustment, why it works, and what the evidence says about its safety. That understanding is genuinely useful to people who've been making decisions based on incomplete information. Pass it on.

Spinal Degeneration — Understanding the Breakdown Before It Breaks You

✦✦✦

What Spinal Degeneration Actually Is and How It Develops

Your spine is not a static structure. It is a living, dynamic system that responds to every load you put on it, every position you hold, every movement you make, and every movement you don't make. It adapts constantly. And when the inputs it receives are consistently poor, the adaptations it makes are consistently destructive. That is spinal degeneration in a nutshell. Not a disease that attacks you from outside. A predictable, internally driven breakdown that follows a clear pattern and almost always starts with the same two things: misalignment and reduced movement.

Most people hear the words "spinal degeneration" and picture an elderly person hunched over a walker. That image is misleading in a dangerous way, because it suggests that degeneration is something that happens to old people, not to you. The reality is that spinal degeneration typically begins in early adulthood. Research using imaging studies has found early degenerative changes in the spines of people in their twenties and thirties who have zero pain and zero awareness that anything is happening. By the time most people receive a formal diagnosis of spinal degeneration, the process has usually been underway for a decade or more.

That's not meant to alarm you. It is meant to reframe how you think about this. Degeneration isn't something that happens to you when you get old. It is something that's been happening to most adults for years already, quietly and without permission, driven by the same entropy that was previously described. The difference between someone whose degeneration progresses slowly and someone whose spine deteriorates rapidly isn't age. It is the quality of care the spine receives over time.

Understanding how degeneration actually develops, stage by stage, changes everything about how you respond to it.

The process starts with what chiropractors and researchers call spinal dysfunction, which is the combination of misalignment and restricted joint movement that previous chapters have described in detail. When a vertebral segment loses its normal motion and shifts slightly out of its optimal position, the mechanical load on the surrounding structures changes. The disc at that level starts receiving uneven pressure. Instead of being compressed and decompressed symmetrically as the joint moves through its full range, the disc gets loaded more heavily on one side than the other. Over time, this uneven loading causes the disc to lose hydration faster on the overloaded side. The disc begins to thin. Its ability to absorb shock decreases. The vertebrae above and below it start to move closer together.

As the disc thins, the space available for the nerve roots that exit the spine at that level gets smaller. The intervertebral foramen, which is the opening through which the nerve root passes, narrows. The nerve root starts to experience compression that it wasn't designed to tolerate chronically. Nerve function at that level begins to deteriorate in the subtle, quiet way that was previously described. And the body, sensing instability in that area, responds the only way it knows how. It tries to stabilize the joint by laying down extra bone. These bony growths are called osteophytes, or more commonly, bone spurs. They are not a malfunction. They are the body's attempt to compensate for a structural problem it can't fully solve on its own. But the compensation creates its own problems. Bone spurs can grow into the nerve spaces, compress the spinal canal, and cause the very nerve irritation the body was trying to protect against.

This progression has been organized into stages that help clinicians and patients understand where they are in the process. Stage one is the dysfunction phase. The joints are restricted and misaligned, but the structural changes are minimal. There may be some mild disc changes beginning, but the bones themselves look mostly normal on imaging. Most people in stage one have no pain at all. This is the stage where intervention is most powerful and where the most complete recovery is possible. Stage two involves more significant disc thinning, early bone spur formation, and measurable narrowing of the nerve spaces. Some people begin to experience intermittent pain or stiffness at this stage, though many still feel nothing. Stage three shows advanced disc degeneration, significant bone spur formation, possible fusion of adjacent vertebrae, and more pronounced nerve compression. Pain is more common at this stage, though even here, some people remain surprisingly asymptomatic. Stage four represents severe structural breakdown with significant loss of disc height, extensive bone spur formation, and potentially severe nerve compromise.

The critical point in all of this is that stages one and two are where the game is won or lost. If the dysfunction driving the degeneration gets addressed at these stages, the progression can be halted and partially reversed. If it doesn't, the process continues compounding, and the options available at stage three or four are significantly more limited than they would have been earlier. This is why waiting for pain before taking action is such a costly strategy. Pain doesn't show up reliably until the process is already well advanced. By the time your back is screaming at you, your spine has been quietly breaking down for years.

A hypothetical scenario makes this concrete. Think about a 38-year-old graphic designer named Tom. He's been sitting at a workstation for ten years, spending six to eight hours a day with his head slightly forward and his lower back rounded away from his chair. He's never had serious back pain. He occasionally feels stiff in the morning, but it goes away after he moves around. He'd describe himself as healthy. If Tom got a spinal X-ray today, there's a significant probability that it would show early degenerative changes at his lower cervical spine and lumbar spine, consistent with stage one or early stage two degeneration. Not because anything dramatic happened to him. Because ten years of poor mechanical loading has been slowly and silently doing what poor mechanical loading always does. Tom doesn't know this because nobody has told him to look. And every year he doesn't look, the process continues. This is a hypothetical example, but it reflects what clinicians see in spinal imaging studies of working adults with sedentary occupations every single day.

Knowing the stages gives you something genuinely useful: a map. You can find out where you are on that map with a proper spinal assessment and imaging. And once you know where you are, you can make informed decisions about what to do about it. That is a completely different position to be in than the one most people occupy, which is simply waiting to see what hurts next.

The Posture-Degeneration Connection — How You Hold Yourself Is Destroying Your Spine

Posture is not about looking confident or standing up straight for a photo. It is a mechanical reality with structural consequences that compound over years into permanent changes in your spine. The way you hold your body for hours every day is either loading your spinal structures within their designed tolerances or loading them outside of those tolerances. There is no middle ground, and the difference between the two determines how fast your spine degenerates.

The human spine was designed to carry load in a specific configuration. From the side, a healthy spine has three natural curves. A gentle forward curve in the neck called the cervical lordosis. A gentle backward curve in the mid-back called the thoracic kyphosis. And a gentle forward curve in the lower back called the lumbar lordosis. These curves aren't cosmetic. They're engineering. They distribute the compressive load of gravity and movement across the entire spine rather than concentrating it at specific points. When those curves are present and properly maintained, the spine handles the demands of daily life remarkably well. When those curves are lost or exaggerated, the load distribution breaks down, and specific segments of the spine start absorbing far more force than they were designed to handle.

Forward head posture is the most widespread and arguably the most damaging postural problem in modern populations. It is what happens when the head drifts forward of the shoulders, which is the natural consequence of looking at screens that are positioned at or below eye level for hours at a time. The human head weighs between ten and twelve pounds in a neutral position, balanced directly over the shoulders. For every inch it moves forward from that neutral position, the effective load on the cervical spine increases dramatically. At two inches forward, the load roughly doubles. At four inches forward, which is extremely common in people who use phones and laptops regularly, the cervical spine is managing the equivalent of nearly sixty pounds of compressive force. For hours. Every day. Over years.

That kind of chronic overloading accelerates disc degeneration in the cervical spine faster than almost any other single factor. The discs at the lower cervical levels, particularly C5-C6 and C6-C7, bear the brunt of this load and are consistently the most commonly degenerated levels in adults who work at desks or use handheld devices extensively. The muscles at the back of the neck become chronically overloaded trying to hold the head up against that increased effective weight. They develop trigger points, areas of sustained contraction that refer pain into the head, shoulders, and upper back. The joints at the front of the cervical spine get compressed while the joints at the back get stretched. The normal cervical lordosis starts to flatten or reverse. And once that curve is lost, the disc degeneration accelerates because the load distribution the curve was providing is gone.

Rounded shoulders compound the problem throughout the thoracic spine. When the shoulders roll forward, the thoracic kyphosis increases beyond its normal range. The discs in the mid-back get compressed at the front and stretched at the back, which is the opposite of their designed load distribution. The muscles between the shoulder blades become chronically lengthened and weakened. The chest muscles shorten. Breathing becomes shallower because the thoracic expansion needed for full inhalation is mechanically restricted by the rounded posture. And the nerve roots exiting the thoracic spine, which serve the organs of the chest and abdomen as previously described, start to experience the same kind of compression and irritation that the cervical roots experience from forward head posture.

The lower back has its own postural crisis. Prolonged sitting flattens the lumbar lordosis. The lower back rounds instead of maintaining its natural inward curve. The discs at L4-L5 and L5-S1, which are already the most heavily loaded segments in the entire spine due to their position at the base of the column, get compressed asymmetrically. The posterior disc wall, which is the part of the disc closest to the spinal cord and nerve roots, comes under increased tension. This is the mechanism behind the disc bulges and herniations that are so common in adults who sit for prolonged periods. The disc isn't failing randomly. It's failing at the point where years of postural loading have repeatedly stressed it beyond its structural limits.

Here is what makes this particularly important to understand. Posture isn't just a problem when you're at your desk. The postural patterns you develop from hours of daily screen use become your default patterns. Your muscles adapt to the shortened and lengthened positions they're held in most often. Your nervous system starts to register those positions as normal. Your joints adapt to the ranges of motion they're actually using rather than the ranges they were designed for. Over months and years, the structural changes that were initially postural become architectural. The curves change. The disc heights change. The bone remodels around the loads it's receiving. What started as a posture problem becomes a structural problem. And structural problems are significantly harder to reverse than postural ones.

The good news is that posture is one of the most modifiable risk factors for spinal degeneration, particularly in the earlier stages. Small corrections made consistently produce measurable structural benefits over time. The spine responds to mechanical input. Give it better input, and it adapts in a better direction. The specific corrections that matter most are straightforward, and they don't require expensive equipment or hours of your time. They require awareness and repetition.

Start with your workstation. Your monitor should be at eye level, so your gaze is horizontal, not angled downward. If you use a laptop, get an external keyboard and raise the screen to eye level. Your chair should support the natural curve of your lower back. If it doesn't, place a small, rolled towel or a lumbar support cushion at the curve of your lower back, positioned at the level of your belt line. Your feet should be flat on the floor. Your ears should sit directly over your shoulders when you're seated. Check these five points right now if you're at a desk. If more than two of them are off, your workstation is actively accelerating spinal degeneration every hour you spend at it.

For your phone, the single most effective change is to bring the phone up to eye level instead of dropping your head to look at it. This one habit, applied consistently, eliminates the forward head load that's the primary driver of cervical degeneration in younger adults. It feels awkward at first because the old pattern is deeply ingrained. Within two weeks of consistent practice, it becomes the default. The cervical spine notices the difference in compressive load almost immediately.

For sleeping, the position that protects the spine best for most people is side lying with a pillow that keeps the head in a neutral position, meaning the ear is level with the shoulder, not tilted up or down. A pillow between the knees keeps the hips and lower back in a neutral alignment. Stomach sleeping is the worst position for the cervical spine because it requires the neck to be rotated to one side for the entire duration of sleep, which applies sustained rotational load to the cervical joints and discs for hours at a time. If you're a stomach sleeper, transitioning away from it is one of the most impactful structural changes you can make for your cervical spine's long-term health.

Can Degeneration Be Reversed? An Honest, Evidence-Based Answer

This is the question most people are quietly carrying when they pick up a book like this. And it deserves a straight answer rather than vague reassurance or deflating pessimism.

The honest answer has three parts, and which part applies to you depends on where you are in the degenerative process.

THE FOUR STAGES OF SPINAL DECAY

STAGE 1

NORMAL

Spine is aligned and healthy.

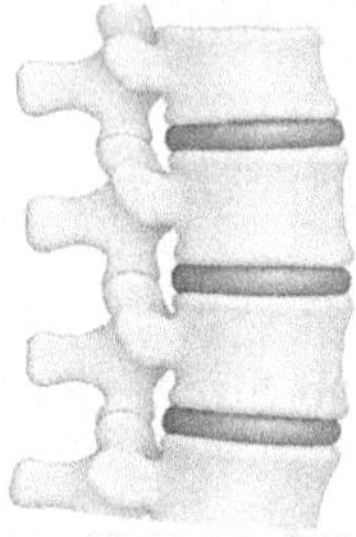

STAGE 2

EARLY DECAY

Minor misalignments and disc weakening begin.

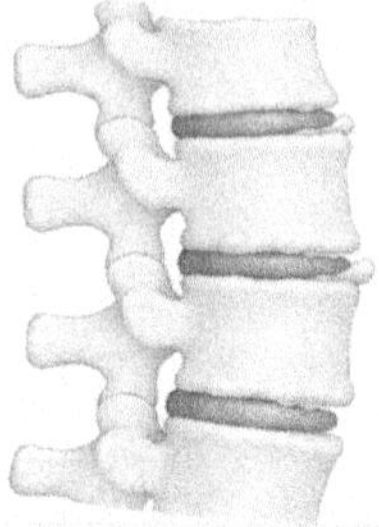

STAGE 3

ADVANCED DECAY

Disc degeneration, bone changes, and misalignments increase.

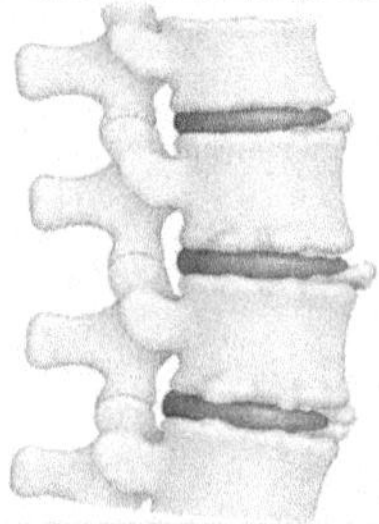

STAGE 4

SEVERE DECAY

Significant bone changes, disc deterioration, and severe misalignments.

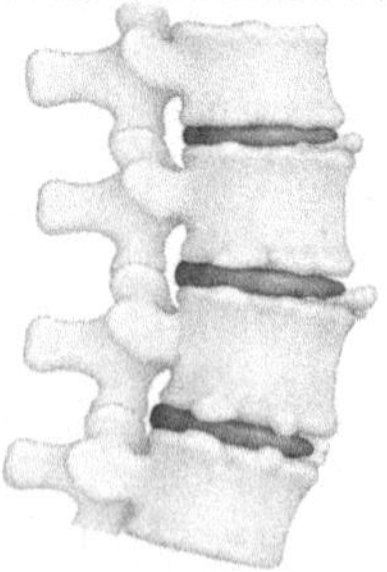

First, some forms of degeneration can be partially reversed. Disc hydration and height can improve when the mechanical loading that was causing the disc to degenerate is corrected, and the joint begins moving properly again. Discs are living tissue. They respond to improved mechanical conditions. Research using serial MRI imaging has shown measurable improvements in disc height and hydration in patients who received consistent chiropractic care combined with targeted rehabilitation over a period of months. This isn't universal, and it isn't dramatic in advanced cases. But it is real, and it happens more reliably in earlier stages of degeneration when the disc tissue still has enough structural integrity to respond to improved conditions.

Bone spurs are not reversible once they've formed. Bone that has been laid down doesn't disappear with conservative care. However, bone spurs that aren't actively compressing nerve tissue often cause no symptoms at all. The goal in managing them isn't to make them disappear. It's to prevent them from growing further by eliminating the mechanical instability that caused the body to lay them down in the first place. Correct the alignment, restore the movement, stabilize the segment with proper muscular support, and the stimulus for further bone spur formation is reduced significantly.

Second, degeneration can be halted. This is perhaps the most practically important part of the answer, because it applies to a much broader range of people than partial reversal does. Even in cases where the structural changes are too advanced to meaningfully reverse, the progression of those changes can be stopped. The research on this is consistent. People who receive regular spinal care, maintain good spinal alignment, move regularly, and support their spinal health with appropriate exercise show significantly slower rates of degenerative progression compared to people who don't. The breakdown doesn't have to keep accelerating. It can be stopped. And stopping the progression of a degenerative process is enormously valuable because every year that passes without further deterioration is a year that quality of life, function, and options for management are preserved.

Third, all stages of degeneration can be managed far more effectively than most people realize. Management doesn't mean masking symptoms with medication. It means reducing the nerve irritation that degenerated structures are producing, improving the function of the joints and muscles around the degenerated area, and maintaining the quality of life and physical function that the degeneration has been threatening. People with stage three and even stage four degeneration regularly experience dramatic improvements in pain, mobility, and daily function through consistent chiropractic care, targeted exercise, and lifestyle modifications. They don't get a new spine. But they get a spine that works significantly better than it did before, and a quality of life that reflects that improvement in ways that matter enormously day to day.

The variable that determines which of these three outcomes is achievable for any individual is the stage of degeneration and how long it's been present. Earlier is always better. Stage one degeneration in a 35-year-old who starts consistent care has a genuinely high probability of partial reversal and complete halting of progression. Stage three degeneration in a 60-year-old who has never had their spine addressed is a different conversation, but it's still very much a conversation worth having, because the management outcomes available even at that stage are far better than the continued decline that comes from doing nothing.

The other critical variable is what you do between appointments. A chiropractor can restore motion to restricted joints and reduce nerve interference during your appointment. But you spend the other twenty-three hours of each day either supporting that work or undoing it. The exercises, the posture corrections, the movement habits, the sleep position, the workstation setup: all of these determine how well the improvements from care hold between sessions and how quickly the spine responds to treatment. The people who get the best outcomes from care for spinal degeneration are consistently the ones who treat their appointments as one piece of a broader daily commitment to their spine, not as the whole solution.

What you should do right now, if you haven't already, is get a spinal X-ray or a comprehensive spinal assessment from a chiropractor who can evaluate both the structural and functional state of your spine. This gives you actual information rather than guesswork. You'll know which stage of degeneration, if any, is present. You'll know which segments are most affected. You'll know what the nerve pathways at those levels are connected to. And you'll have a clear starting point for a care plan that's built around your specific spine rather than a generic protocol. That specificity is what produces real results, and it starts with knowing exactly what you're working with.

The Role of Inflammation — Why Your Spine Is Constantly Under Fire

Inflammation gets a lot of attention in health conversations, and most of it focuses on diet, exercise, and lifestyle. Those factors matter. But there's a source of chronic inflammation that almost nobody talks about in this context, and it sits inside your spine.

When a spinal joint is misaligned and moving improperly, the tissues surrounding that joint respond the same way any tissue responds to mechanical stress it wasn't designed to handle. They become inflamed. The joint capsule, the ligaments, the disc tissue, and the adjacent muscles all produce inflammatory chemicals in response to the chronic abnormal loading. This is a local inflammatory response, and in the short term, it's appropriate. Inflammation is part of the repair process. The problem is that when the mechanical cause of the inflammation, the misalignment and restricted movement, isn't corrected, the inflammatory response never gets to finish its job. It becomes chronic. And chronic inflammation is a fundamentally different animal from acute inflammation.

Acute inflammation is purposeful and time limited. It brings resources to an injured area, does its work, and resolves. Chronic inflammation is a sustained, low-grade process that damages the very tissues it was supposed to repair. In the spine, chronic joint inflammation accelerates disc degeneration by breaking down the proteoglycans that give disc tissue its ability to hold water and resist compression. It damages the cartilage lining the facet joints, the small joints at the back of each vertebral segment that guide and limit spinal movement. It irritates the nerve roots passing through the inflamed area, producing the kind of low-grade nerve irritation that shows up as the diffuse, hard-to-locate pain that many people describe as their back being "generally sore" rather than hurting in one specific spot.

The cycle that this creates is one of the most important concepts in understanding why spinal degeneration progresses the way it does. Misalignment produces inflammation. Inflammation damages disc and joint tissue. Damaged tissue leads to more instability and further misalignment. More misalignment produces more inflammation. The cycle feeds itself, and without intervention that breaks the mechanical cause, it keeps accelerating. This is entropy operating through inflammation, and it's running in the background of millions of people's spines right now.

Spinal adjustments interrupt this cycle at the mechanical level. By restoring proper motion and alignment to the affected segments, they reduce the abnormal mechanical stress that's driving the inflammatory response. When the joint starts moving properly and loading more symmetrically, the stimulus for chronic inflammation decreases. The inflammatory process can begin to resolve rather than sustaining itself indefinitely. This is one of the reasons that people with chronic spinal pain often notice not just reduced pain but a qualitative change in how the area feels after consistent care. The deep, constant ache that comes from chronic inflammation feels different from the sharper, more mechanical pain of restricted movement. When both resolve, the change is noticeable and significant.

Nutrition plays a direct supporting role in managing spinal inflammation, and it's specific enough to be worth addressing clearly. Certain foods consistently promote inflammatory signaling throughout the body, including refined carbohydrates, processed vegetable oils high in omega-6 fatty acids, added sugar, and ultra-processed foods. These don't just cause systemic inflammation in a vague, general way. They elevate specific inflammatory markers including C-reactive protein and interleukin-6 that directly influence the inflammatory environment in spinal joints and discs. Reducing these foods and replacing them with anti-inflammatory alternatives, primarily vegetables, fruits, fatty fish, olive oil, nuts, and whole grains, reduces the systemic inflammatory load that the spine is operating in. The spine still needs mechanical correction. But doing that correction in a body with lower systemic inflammation produces better and faster results than doing it in a body where the inflammatory fire is being constantly refueled by diet.

Three specific nutritional changes produce the biggest reduction in spinal inflammation for most people. First, replace refined vegetable oils like soybean, corn, and sunflower oil with olive oil or avocado oil for cooking. This shifts the omega-6 to omega-3 ratio in the diet toward a range that supports anti-inflammatory signaling rather than pro-inflammatory signaling. Second, add fatty fish to your diet at least twice a week. Salmon, sardines, mackerel, and herring are all high in eicosapentaenoic acid (EPA) and docosahexaenoic acid (DHA), the omega-3 fatty acids that directly reduce the production of inflammatory prostaglandins. If fish isn't practical, a high-quality fish oil supplement providing at least two grams of combined EPA and DHA daily produces measurable reductions in inflammatory markers within four to six weeks. Third, reduce added sugar to below twenty-five grams per day. Sugar is one of the most potent dietary drivers of systemic inflammation, and most people consume two to three times this amount without realizing it. Reading labels and identifying the primary sources of added sugar in your current diet, then replacing those sources with whole food alternatives, is the single dietary change that produces the most consistent reduction in systemic inflammatory markers in the shortest time.

Movement is the other critical tool for managing spinal inflammation, and its mechanism is different from nutrition's. Regular, low-to-moderate intensity movement reduces inflammation through several pathways. It improves blood flow to spinal structures, which helps clear inflammatory byproducts from the joint environment. It promotes the production of anti-inflammatory cytokines through muscle contraction. It drives the compression-decompression cycle that keeps spinal discs hydrated and nourished. And it maintains the joint mobility that prevents the stagnation that allows chronic inflammation to take hold.

"Movement is improvement."

—Dr. Moshe Feldenkrais,
Renowned engineer and Physical Therapist

The specific type of movement matters. High-impact, high-intensity exercise during an acute inflammatory flare can worsen things. But consistent, daily, low-to-moderate movement, walking, swimming, cycling, yoga, or the spinal mobility work described in detail earlier, is one of the most powerful anti-inflammatory tools available and one of the most consistently underused ones.

Your Spine at Every Age — What to Expect and What to Do About It

Spinal health isn't a single conversation. It is a different conversation at age 25 than it is at 45, and a different one again at age 65. The challenges change. The priorities shift. The strategies that matter most evolve as the body changes. Understanding what's happening in your spine at your specific life stage, and what actions make the biggest difference right now, is far more useful than generic advice that doesn't account for where you actually are.

In your twenties and early thirties, the spine is at its most resilient and most adaptable. Disc tissue is well-hydrated, bone density is at or near its peak, and the body's capacity to respond to good care is at its highest. This is also the decade where the habits and postures that will drive degeneration for the next forty years are being established. The person who spends their twenties sitting for eight hours a day in poor posture, rarely moving their spine through its full range, and never getting it assessed is laying the structural groundwork for stage two or three degeneration by their mid-forties. The person who establishes good spinal habits, gets assessed, and addresses any early dysfunction in this decade is building a structural foundation that pays dividends for decades.

The most important actions in this age group are preventive. Get a baseline spinal assessment even if nothing hurts. Establish a daily spinal mobility practice. Audit and correct your workstation and phone habits before they've had decades to compound. If you play sports or do any kind of repetitive physical activity, get your spine checked regularly for the asymmetric loading patterns that sports and repetitive work create. The spine is most responsive to correction in this decade, and the return on investment for care at this stage is higher than at any other point in life.

In your late thirties and forties, the picture changes. Disc hydration begins to decline naturally as part of the aging process, even in healthy spines. The cumulative effects of the postural and movement habits from the previous decade start to show up on imaging, even in people who feel relatively fine. This is the decade when most people first start to notice the symptoms that signal early to mid-stage degeneration. Morning stiffness that takes longer to clear. Neck tension that doesn't fully go away. Lower back aches that come on after long drives or desk sessions. These aren't random. They are the first functional signals of structural changes that have been building for years.

This is also the decade where the gap between people who take action and people who don't starts to widen significantly. The person who starts consistent chiropractic care, corrects their posture, and builds a regular movement practice in their late thirties or early forties can halt degeneration at its current stage and in many cases partially reverse the early changes. The person who dismisses the symptoms as normal aging and does nothing watches the process continue compounding. The specific priorities for this age group are corrective. Address any existing subluxations and degeneration with a structured care plan. Build the core and spinal stabilizer strength that reduces mechanical stress on the discs and joints. Establish the postural corrections that change the loading environment the spine operates in. And commit to regular maintenance adjustments, ideally monthly, to keep the spine moving properly as the natural age-related changes in disc hydration begin.

In your fifties and sixties, the conversation shifts again. Disc height loss is more pronounced. Bone density begins to decline, particularly in women following menopause. The range of motion available in the spine decreases as ligaments and joint capsules lose some of their elasticity. Nerve compression from degenerated structures becomes more common, and the symptoms it produces are more likely to be present and more likely to be significant. This is the decade when many people receive their first formal diagnosis of spinal degeneration, often after an imaging study done for some other reason reveals changes that have been building for twenty years.

The most important thing to understand about spinal health in this decade is that the diagnosis is not the end of the story. It is the beginning of a more informed chapter. Knowing what stage of degeneration is present, which segments are most affected, and what the nerve implications are gives you the information you need to make genuinely effective decisions about care. Chiropractic techniques are adapted for the changes in tissue quality that come with this age group. Gentler methods, including flexion-distraction therapy, which uses a specialized table to gently decompress the lumbar discs and restore motion without high-velocity thrusting, are particularly effective for lumbar degeneration with nerve involvement in this population. The goals shift from reversal to management and preservation of function, and those goals are entirely achievable with the right care plan.

Exercise becomes even more critical in this decade. Bone density responds to load-bearing exercise, and maintaining bone density reduces the risk of the vertebral compression fractures that become more common as degeneration advances. Resistance training two to three times per week, focusing on functional movements that load the spine in its designed ranges, is one of the most evidence-supported interventions for maintaining spinal health and overall physical function in the fifties and sixties. Combined with regular spinal care, it produces outcomes that consistently exceed what either approach produces alone.

In your seventies and beyond, the primary goals are maintaining function, preserving independence, and managing pain effectively without relying on interventions that create new problems. Spinal degeneration at this stage is typically more advanced, but the body's capacity to respond to good care doesn't disappear. Research consistently shows that older adults who receive regular chiropractic care maintain better spinal mobility, experience less pain, fall less frequently due to improved balance and proprioception, and report higher quality of life than comparable adults who don't.[31][32] The techniques used are gentler, the pace of change is slower, and the expectations are appropriately calibrated. But the direction of change, toward better function and less pain, is the same regardless of age.

Balance work becomes critically important in this age group. The proprioceptive input from spinal joints described previously as essential for brain-body coordination declines with advancing degeneration, and this decline directly contributes to the increased fall risk that becomes a serious health concern for older adults. Regular spinal adjustments that keep the remaining mobile segments moving properly, combined with specific balance and coordination exercises, directly address this risk. A simple daily practice of standing on one foot for thirty seconds on each side, progressing to doing this with eyes closed as balance improves, is a specific, evidence-supported exercise that improves proprioceptive function and reduces fall risk in older adults. It takes two minutes and can be done anywhere.

What to Do With Everything You Now Know

Spinal degeneration follows a predictable pattern. It starts with misalignment and restricted movement, progresses through stages of disc thinning, bone spur formation, and nerve compression, and is driven forward by chronic inflammation and the entropy that works on every unattended structure over time. It starts silently, long before pain appears, and it compounds quietly for years before most people know it's happening.

The most important thing this chapter gives you is a framework for action that's based on where you actually are rather than on waiting to see where you end up. Every stage of degeneration responds to the right care. Earlier stages respond more dramatically. Later stages still respond meaningfully. And the daily choices you make about posture, movement, nutrition, and spinal care are either slowing this process down or letting it run unchecked. There's no neutral position. That principle has been consistent throughout this entire book, and it's as true for spinal degeneration as it is for every other aspect of the entropy that's been working on your body since the day you were born.

Three specific actions to take before you move into the next chapter.

First, book a spinal X-ray or comprehensive spinal assessment this week. Ask your chiropractor specifically to evaluate you for signs of degeneration and to tell you which stage, if any, is present at each spinal level. Ask which segments show the most restriction, where the nerve compression risk is highest, and what a realistic care plan looks like for your specific findings. This one step replaces guesswork with actual information, and actual information is the only foundation on which a genuinely effective plan can be built.

Second, audit your three highest-risk posture environments today. Your desk, your car, and your phone position. Use the specific corrections described in this chapter and make at least one concrete change in each environment before you go to sleep tonight. Do not wait until you've had time to do it perfectly. One real change today beats a perfect plan that starts next week.

Third, add the two anti-inflammatory nutritional changes that are most practical for your current diet. If you cook with refined vegetable oils, replace them with olive oil starting with your next meal. If you don't eat fatty fish regularly, add it twice this week or start a fish oil supplement at the dose described in this chapter. These aren't dramatic dietary overhauls. They're specific, targeted changes that reduce the systemic inflammatory environment your spine is operating in and support every other element of the care plan you're building.

Movement Is Medicine — Why Staying Still Is Slowly Killing You

✦✦✦

The Biology of Movement — Why Your Body Was Designed to Keep Moving

Your spine doesn't have its own blood supply the way your muscles or organs do. That single fact changes everything about how you need to think about keeping it healthy.

Most tissues in your body get their nutrients delivered directly through blood vessels. Blood flows in, drops off oxygen and nutrients, picks up waste products, and flows back out. Clean, efficient, continuous. But your spinal discs work differently. They don't have that direct blood supply. Instead, they rely on a process called imbibition, which is essentially the disc acting like a sponge. When load is applied to the disc and then released, it compresses and then expands, drawing in fluid and nutrients from the surrounding tissue. Compress, release, absorb. Compress, release, absorb. That cycle is how your discs stay hydrated, nourished, and structurally resilient. And the only thing that drives that cycle is movement.

Stop moving, and the disc stops imbibing.

This is not a minor detail. It is the biological reason why a sedentary lifestyle is one of the most powerful accelerators of spinal degeneration available. When you sit still for hours, your discs are under sustained, relatively static compression. The imbibition cycle slows dramatically. The disc loses hydration. It loses height. It becomes stiffer and less able to absorb the shock loads that daily life puts through the spine. Over months and years, what started as a simple lack of movement compounds into the kind of structural disc changes that were described in detail earlier. Not because anything violent happened. Because the spine was starved of the one input it needs most: motion.

The facet joints of the spine, which are the small, paired joints at the back of each vertebral segment, have a similar dependency on movement for their health. Joint cartilage is nourished by synovial fluid, and synovial fluid gets distributed across the joint surface through movement. A joint that doesn't move regularly develops areas of cartilage that are chronically undernourished. Those areas become thinner, less resilient, and more prone to the kind of wear that eventually shows up as arthritis and bone spur formation. This is the same mechanism behind why people who immobilize a joint after an injury are encouraged to begin gentle, controlled movement as soon as safely possible. Immobilization protects the injury in the short term but starves the joint of what it needs to heal and stay healthy.

Movement also feeds the nervous system in a way that's just as important as the nutritional effect on the discs and joints. As previously described, the joints of the spine are packed with mechanoreceptors, sensory cells that fire signals to the brain every time the joint moves. That constant stream of sensory input is what keeps the brain accurately informed about the state of the body, what keeps motor control precise, what keeps balance calibrated, and what keeps the brain itself stimulated and alert. When the spine stops moving, that sensory stream drops. The brain receives less input from one of its richest sources of information. Motor control becomes less precise. Balance deteriorates slightly. Cognitive sharpness dims in ways that are subtle but measurable. Movement isn't just good for your back. It is a direct input into brain function, and reducing it has consequences that extend well beyond the spine itself.

The research on this is striking. Studies examining the effects of prolonged sitting on spinal health have found measurable increases in disc pressure, reduced muscle activation in the deep spinal stabilizers, and changes in lumbar curve geometry within as little as twenty to thirty minutes of continuous sitting.[33][34] These aren't long-term effects from years of sedentary behavior. They're acute, immediate responses to staying still. Now multiply those effects by six, eight, or ten hours of sitting per day, five days a week, fifty-two weeks a year, for a decade or two, and the cumulative picture becomes clear. Entropy doesn't need a dramatic cause. It just needs enough time and enough stillness to do its work.

Here is what makes this particularly relevant for the way most people live right now. The modern work environment is structured around sitting. The modern entertainment environment is structured around sitting. The modern transportation environment is structured around sitting. A significant portion of the population spends the vast majority of their waking hours in a posture that loads the spine statically, reduces disc nutrition, starves the facet joints of synovial circulation, and drops the sensory input to the brain that movement would otherwise be providing. And then those same people wonder why their backs hurt, why they feel stiff and tired, and why their bodies seem to be aging faster than they should. The answer isn't mysterious. The spine was built to move. When it doesn't, it breaks down. That is not a theory. It is biology.

The good news is that the biological requirement for movement doesn't demand marathon training or hours in a gym. The imbibition cycle that feeds your discs responds to any movement that loads and unloads the spine rhythmically. Walking does it. Simple spinal mobility exercises do it. Even standing up from your desk and shifting your weight does it. The threshold for keeping the spine nutritionally supplied through movement is not high. But it does require consistency, because the disc's nutritional cycle depends on repeated, regular input throughout the day rather than one long bout of movement followed by hours of stillness.

Think about what a typical Tuesday looks like for a hypothetical 43-year-old project coordinator named Lisa. She wakes up, sits at the breakfast table for fifteen minutes, drives forty minutes to work, sits at her desk for four hours, drives to a lunch meeting, sits through that meeting for an hour, drives back, sits at her desk for another three hours, drives home, sits through dinner, and then sits on the couch for two hours before bed. On a generous count, Lisa's spine is in sustained static compression for somewhere between ten and twelve hours of her waking day. She moves between sitting positions, but she rarely takes her spine through any meaningful range of motion. She doesn't think of herself as sedentary because she's busy and active in terms of her mental output. But her spine is operating in the nutritional equivalent of a drought. This is a hypothetical scenario, but it describes the daily reality of a very large number of working adults. And it's exactly the kind of daily pattern that makes movement not a nice-to-have but a genuine biological necessity.

The principle that ties all of this together is one that runs through every chapter of this book. Your body is either moving toward health or moving toward breakdown. There is no standing still, and in the case of the spine, that principle is almost literally true. Standing still, or more accurately sitting still, is one of the most direct paths toward the kind of spinal degeneration that eventually becomes impossible to ignore. Movement is the counterforce. It is the input the spine needs to stay nourished, mobile, and structurally sound. And understanding that movement is a biological requirement rather than an optional extra is the foundation for everything that follows in this chapter.

The Difference Between Exercise and Therapeutic Movement

Not all movement is created equal when your spine is involved. This is one of the most important distinctions in this entire chapter and getting it wrong can make things significantly worse rather than better.

General exercise is movement designed to improve cardiovascular fitness, build muscle strength, increase endurance, or burn calories. These are all legitimate and valuable goals. But general exercise is not designed with your specific spinal mechanics in mind. It doesn't account for which segments of your spine are restricted, which muscles are compensating for those restrictions, or which movement patterns have become distorted by years of poor posture and accumulated dysfunction. When you take a spine that has existing misalignments, restricted segments, and compensatory muscle patterns, and you load it heavily through general exercise without addressing those underlying issues first, you're not just exercising. You're loading a compromised structure under increased demand. And loading a compromised structure under increased demand accelerates the breakdown of that structure.

This is why some people find that their back pain gets worse after starting a new exercise program. It is not that exercise is bad for the spine.

It is that exercise performed through dysfunctional movement patterns, with restricted joints and unbalanced muscle activation, reinforces and compounds the dysfunction rather than correcting it. The body adapts to the demands placed on it. If those demands are placed through broken movement patterns, the body gets better at moving through broken patterns. That is not progress. That is a deeper rut.

Therapeutic movement is different. It is specific, intentional, and designed around the actual state of your spine rather than a generic fitness goal. It targets the joints and movement patterns that need to be restored, activates the muscles that have been inhibited by spinal dysfunction, and progressively reloads the spine in ways that support healing rather than accelerating breakdown. The goal of therapeutic movement isn't to get fit. It is to restore the mechanical function of the spine so that the spine can handle the demands of daily life and general exercise without continuing to break down.

There are four specific categories of therapeutic movement that matter most for spinal health and understanding what each one does and why it's necessary gives you a framework for building a movement practice that actually works.

The first category is spinal mobility work. This is movement designed to restore the full, normal range of motion to each region of the spine. The cervical spine should be able to rotate approximately 80 degrees in each direction, flex forward until the chin approaches the chest, and extend backward comfortably. The thoracic spine should be able to rotate, flex, and extend through ranges that allow the ribcage to expand fully with breathing and the upper body to rotate freely during walking and reaching. The lumbar spine should be able to flex, extend, and side-bend through its designed ranges without pain or restriction. When any of these ranges are limited, the segments above and below compensate by moving more than they should, which overloads those segments and accelerates their degeneration. Mobility work restores these ranges progressively, reducing the compensatory overload on adjacent segments and improving the overall mechanical efficiency of the spine.

The second category is deep stabilizer activation. The spine is stabilized by two layers of muscle. The outer layer consists of the larger, more powerful muscles like the erector spinae, the latissimus dorsi, and the gluteus maximus. These are the muscles most people think of when they think about back strength. But the inner layer, which includes the multifidus, the transversus abdominis, the pelvic floor, and the deep hip rotators, is the layer that actually provides the moment-to-moment stability that protects the spine during movement. These muscles are small, slow-twitch, and designed for endurance rather than power. They are also the muscles that shut down first when spinal dysfunction is present. When a segment subluxates or becomes restricted, the deep stabilizers at that level become inhibited. The outer muscles compensate, but they're not designed for the constant, precise stabilization role. They fatigue, they develop trigger points, and they create the kind of diffuse, persistent aching that most people describe as "muscle tension" in their back. Therapeutic movement that specifically targets and reactivates the deep stabilizers addresses the root of this problem rather than just stretching the outer muscles that are compensating for it.

The third category is movement pattern retraining. Years of sitting in poor posture, moving with restricted spinal segments, and compensating for dysfunction create deeply ingrained movement patterns that the nervous system has registered as normal. Bending from the lower back instead of hinging from the hips. Reaching overhead by extending the lumbar spine instead of mobilizing the thoracic spine and shoulder. Walking with a reduced arm swing because the thoracic rotation needed for that swing has been lost. These patterns feel natural because they're familiar, but they're loading the spine incorrectly with every repetition.

Movement pattern retraining teaches the nervous system new patterns that distribute load correctly across the spine and reduce the mechanical stress on the segments that have been absorbing more than their share. This isn't complicated, but it requires conscious repetition until the new pattern becomes the default.

The fourth category is progressive loading. Once mobility is restored, deep stabilizers are activated, and movement patterns are corrected, the spine needs to be progressively loaded to rebuild the structural strength and resilience that degeneration and disuse have reduced. This means gradually increasing the mechanical demands placed on the spine through exercises that load it in its corrected alignment and through its restored range of motion. Deadlifts, squats, carries, and loaded carries done with proper form and appropriate load are among the most effective tools for rebuilding spinal strength. But the word "progressive" is critical. Starting with loads that are too heavy, too soon, before mobility and movement patterns have been restored, is exactly the mistake that causes exercise to make spinal problems worse rather than better.

The relationship between therapeutic movement and chiropractic care is not competitive. It is synergistic. An adjustment restores motion to restricted joints and reduces nerve interference. Therapeutic movement then takes advantage of that restored motion to rebuild the strength and movement patterns that keep the spine in its corrected state. Without the adjustment, therapeutic movement is being done through a spine that still has mechanical restrictions that limit its range and distort its movement patterns. Without therapeutic movement, the adjustments don't hold as well because the muscular and neuromuscular support that maintains the corrected alignment hasn't been rebuilt. The two approaches together produce outcomes that neither produces as effectively alone. This is why modern chiropractic care increasingly incorporates rehabilitation and movement retraining as core components of the care plan rather than treating the adjustment as the complete intervention.

The distinction between exercise and therapeutic movement also has practical implications for what you do on your own. If you currently exercise regularly, that's genuinely valuable and you shouldn't stop. But if you have existing spinal dysfunction, restricted segments, or any of the degenerative changes described previously, adding therapeutic movement that specifically targets those issues gives your general exercise a foundation to work from rather than a compromised structure to load through. Talk to your chiropractor about which specific therapeutic movements are appropriate for your spinal findings. The answer will be different for someone with cervical degeneration and forward head posture than it will be for someone with lumbar disc thinning and a flattened lordosis. Generic movement advice helps generically. Specific therapeutic movement matched to your specific spinal findings helps specifically, and specific always beats generic when it comes to rehabilitation.

Building a Movement Practice That Protects Your Spine for Life

Consistency beats intensity every single time when it comes to spinal health. Twenty-minute daily movement done seven days a week produces better outcomes than a two-hour session done twice a week. The spine responds to regular, repeated input. The imbibition cycle that feeds the discs needs to happen throughout the day, not just during one concentrated window. The deep stabilizers that protect the spine need to be trained for endurance, not just peak activation. The movement patterns that protect the spine need to be practiced enough times that they become the default, not the exception. All of that requires consistency, and consistency requires a practice that's sustainable in the context of a real, busy life.

The framework below is specific and practical. It's built around three time windows that most people can realistically access without restructuring their entire day. The morning window, the workday window, and the evening window. Each one serves a distinct purpose, and together they create the kind of consistent daily input that keeps the spine healthy over the long term.

The morning window is ten minutes, done before you leave the house. Its purpose is to restore mobility to a spine that has been relatively static during sleep and to activate the deep stabilizers before you load the spine with the demands of the day. Here is the specific sequence, done in order.

Start with ten slow, controlled cat-cow movements on your hands and knees. Inhale as you drop your belly toward the floor and lift your head gently. Exhale as you round your spine toward the ceiling and drop your head. Move slowly, breathing into each position for a full breath cycle before transitioning. This mobilizes the entire lumbar and thoracic spine, stimulates the imbibition cycle in the lumbar discs, and begins activating the deep spinal stabilizers through the controlled co-contraction that the movement requires. Ten repetitions take about ninety seconds.

Follow with ten thoracic rotations in the seated position. Sit on the floor with your legs crossed or on a chair with your feet flat on the floor. Place your hands on your shoulders with your elbows pointing forward. Keeping your hips still, rotate your upper body as far as you comfortably can to the right, hold for two seconds, return to center, and repeat to the left. This specifically targets the thoracic rotation that desk posture consistently reduces, restores the rib cage mobility needed for full breathing, and reduces the compensatory load on the lumbar spine that thoracic stiffness creates. Ten repetitions per side takes about two minutes.

Then do ten chin tucks. Sit or stand tall with your shoulders relaxed. Without tilting your head up or down, draw your chin straight back, as if making a double chin, and hold for three seconds before releasing. This restores the cervical lordosis that forward head posture flattens, activates the deep cervical flexors that support the head's weight properly, and reduces the compressive load on the lower cervical discs. Ten repetitions take about one minute.

Finish the morning sequence with a two-minute dead bug exercise. Lie on your back with your knees bent at 90 degrees and your arms pointing straight toward the ceiling. Slowly extend your right leg out straight while simultaneously lowering your left arm overhead toward the floor, keeping your lower back pressed firmly against the floor throughout. Return to the starting position and repeat on the opposite side. This directly activates the transversus abdominis and multifidus, the two most important deep stabilizers of the lumbar spine, in a way that teaches them to work together to maintain spinal stability during limb movement. This is the movement pattern that protects the lumbar spine during virtually every daily activity and training it first thing in the morning primes it for the demands of the day. Ten repetitions per side takes about two minutes.

The entire morning sequence takes ten minutes. Set your alarm ten minutes earlier than you currently wake up and do this before you check your phone or do anything else. The consistency of doing it first, before the day's demands can crowd it out, is what makes it sustainable.

The workday window is not a structured exercise session. It is a series of brief, regular movement breaks that prevent the sustained static compression that damages discs and shuts down deep stabilizers during prolonged sitting. The specific protocol is this: set a timer on your phone or computer to go off every forty-five minutes during your workday. When it goes off, stand up and do one of the following for two minutes before sitting back down.

Option one: Walk to get a glass of water. The walking itself is the point. It loads the lumbar discs rhythmically, activates the gluteal muscles that support the lumbar spine, and stimulates the thoracic rotation that sitting eliminates. Option two: Stand and do ten slow shoulder rolls backward, then ten slow neck rotations, moving your ear toward your shoulder on each side and holding for three seconds. This directly counteracts the forward shoulder rounding and lateral neck compression that accumulates during desk work. Option three: Stand with your feet hip-width apart and do ten slow hip hinges, pushing your hips back and keeping your spine long and neutral as you hinge forward, then driving your hips forward to return to standing. This reactivates the posterior chain muscles, including the hamstrings and glutes, that become inhibited during prolonged sitting and that are essential for protecting the lumbar spine during lifting and bending.

Rotating through these three options throughout the workday takes a total of about sixteen minutes across an eight-hour workday if done every forty-five minutes. That is sixteen minutes spread across eight hours. It is not a significant time investment. But the cumulative effect on disc nutrition, deep stabilizer activation, and movement pattern maintenance is substantial. The research on movement breaks during sedentary work is consistent: even two-minute breaks every hour significantly reduces the disc pressure buildup, muscle fatigue, and postural deterioration that accumulate during continuous sitting. The breaks don't need to be long. They need to be regular.

The evening window is optional but valuable, particularly for people with existing spinal dysfunction or degeneration. It is five to ten minutes of gentle spinal mobility and soft tissue work done before bed. Its purpose is to decompress structures that have been loaded throughout the day and to shift the nervous system toward the parasympathetic state that supports healing during sleep.

The most effective evening practice for most people combines two elements. The first is a three-minute supine spinal twist. Lie on your back with your knees bent. Let both knees fall slowly to one side while you look in the opposite direction and breathe slowly and deeply in this position for ninety seconds before switching sides. This gently mobilizes the lumbar and thoracic facet joints, releases the hip flexors and piriformis that become shortened during sitting, and activates the parasympathetic nervous system through the combination of gentle movement and slow breathing. The second element is two minutes of legs-up-the-wall. Lie on your back and rest your legs vertically against a wall with your hips close to the baseboard. This position decompresses the lumbar spine, improves venous return from the legs, and is one of the most reliably effective positions for activating the parasympathetic nervous system and reducing the residual sympathetic tone that accumulates during a demanding day.

Beyond these three windows, there are two broader movement habits that make the biggest difference for spinal health over the long term and that deserve specific mention.

The first is daily walking. Not as a workout, though it serves that purpose too. As a spinal health practice. Walking is the most natural, most complete movement the human spine was designed for. It loads the lumbar discs rhythmically through the imbibition cycle. It drives thoracic rotation that keeps the mid-back mobile. It activates the gluteal muscles that are the primary dynamic stabilizers of the lumbar spine. It stimulates the proprioceptive input to the brain that keeps motor control precise and balance calibrated. Thirty minutes of walking at a comfortable pace, done daily, produces benefits for spinal health that no other single activity fully replicates. If you currently don't walk daily, adding this one habit produces more long-term benefit for your spine than almost any other single change you could make. Walk in the morning, at lunch, or in the evening. The timing matters less than the consistency.

The second is swimming or water-based movement, particularly for people with more advanced spinal degeneration or significant pain that limits land-based movement. Water reduces the compressive load on the spine by approximately 90 percent when the body is submerged to shoulder height. This allows people with painful spinal conditions to move their spine through ranges of motion that would be too painful or too risky on land, stimulating the imbibition cycle and maintaining joint mobility without the compressive loading that aggravates degenerated structures. If land-based movement is currently limited by pain, water-based movement is not a lesser alternative. It is a genuinely superior starting point for rebuilding spinal mobility in a way that the spine can tolerate and respond to positively.

One final point about building a sustainable movement practice deserves emphasis. The biggest obstacle to consistency isn't motivation. It is friction. The practices that get done reliably are the ones that are easy to start, don't require special equipment or a trip to the gym, and fit naturally into the structure of the day that already exists. The morning sequence described above requires a floor and ten minutes. The workday breaks require a timer and the willingness to stand up. The evening practice requires a wall and five minutes. None of it requires a gym membership, special clothing, or a significant rearrangement of your schedule. That low barrier to entry is intentional because a simple practice done every day beats a sophisticated program done sporadically every single time.

Your spine was built to move. Every time you move it well and move it consistently, you're pushing back against the entropy that's been working on it since the day you were born. Every time you sit still for hours without a break, you're letting entropy win a little more ground. The choice between those two outcomes isn't made in dramatic moments. It is made in the small, daily decisions about whether to set the timer, stand up, take the walk, and do the ten minutes in the morning. Those decisions compound over months and years into a spine that either holds up or breaks down. The direction is yours to choose.

What to Do Next

Movement is not supplemental to spinal health. It is the mechanism by which the spine receives its nutrition, maintains its structural integrity, feeds the brain the sensory input it depends on, and pushes back against the entropy that's working on it every single day. The right kind of movement, done consistently, is one of the most powerful tools you have. The wrong kind of movement, or no movement at all, accelerates the very breakdown this book has been describing from the first page.

You now have a specific, practical framework for building a daily movement practice that addresses all four categories of therapeutic movement, works within the time constraints of a real life, and compounds into meaningful long-term protection for your spine. The framework isn't complicated. It is consistent. And consistency is the only thing that actually changes anything.

Four specific actions to take before you move on to the next chapter.

First, set your alarm ten minutes earlier starting tomorrow morning and do the morning sequence described in this chapter. Cat-cow, thoracic rotations, chin tucks, dead bugs. In that order, every morning, before you do anything else. Do it for fourteen consecutive days without missing a day. After fourteen days, assess how your spine feels in the morning compared to how it felt before you started. The difference will give you all the motivation you need to continue.

Second, set a recurring timer on your phone for every forty-five minutes during your workday, starting tomorrow. Label it "spine break" so you know exactly what it's for. When it goes off, stand up and do one of the three two-minute movement options described in this chapter before sitting back down. Rotate through the three options so you're not doing the same one repeatedly. Track how many breaks you actually take in a day for the first week. Most people are surprised to find they take fewer than they intended, and that awareness alone drives improvement.

Third, add a thirty-minute walk to your daily routine this week. Pick a specific time slot and put it in your calendar as a recurring appointment. Morning before work, lunch break, or after dinner all work equally well. The specific time matters less than the fact that it's scheduled and protected. Walking is the single highest-return movement investment available for long-term spinal health, and thirty minutes a day is the threshold at which the research consistently shows meaningful benefits.

Fourth, talk to your chiropractor at your next appointment about which specific therapeutic movement categories are most relevant for your current spinal findings. Ask them to show you the two or three exercises that will produce the most benefit for your specific restrictions and degenerative changes. Ask how those exercises fit with your adjustment plan and what progression looks like over the next thirty and sixty days. A movement plan that's tailored to your actual spinal findings is significantly more effective than a generic one, and your chiropractor has the information needed to build that tailored plan. Use it.

It's Not Just About Pain — The Performance Case for Spinal Health

✦✦✦

Why Chiropractic Is Not Just for People in Crisis

Most people think of chiropractic care the same way they think of an emergency room. You go when something is wrong. You stop going when the problem is fixed. You don't think about it in between. That mental model makes sense on the surface, but it's costing people far more than they realize, not just in terms of pain they could avoid, but in terms of performance, energy, and quality of life they're leaving on the table every single day.

Think about how you treat your teeth. You don't wait until a tooth is throbbing before you brush. You don't skip dental cleanings until you're in agony. You maintain your teeth proactively because you understand that maintenance prevents breakdown. The spine deserves exactly the same logic, and the stakes are actually higher, because the spine houses and protects the nervous system that runs your entire body. Yet most people treat it like a car they only take to the mechanic when the engine light comes on.

The shift that needs to happen is a shift in identity. You are not a patient managing a problem. You are a person with a body that either gets maintained or breaks down, and you get to decide which direction it goes. That reframe changes everything about how you approach spinal care, because it moves the conversation from crisis response to performance optimization.

Elite athletes figured this out decades ago. Every NFL team has a chiropractor on staff. So do Olympic programs, NBA franchises, and professional tennis tours. These aren't athletes who are broken. They are athletes who want every possible advantage, and they've learned that a spine that moves freely and a nervous system that communicates without interference means faster reaction times, better coordination, more efficient movement, and faster recovery between training sessions. They are not going to the chiropractor because their back hurts. They are going because their back not hurting isn't enough. They want every system running at full capacity.

You don't have to be a professional athlete to apply that same thinking to your own life. Whether your performance goals involve running a 5K race, keeping up with your kids or grandkids, sitting through a full workday without your neck screaming at you, or simply having enough energy at the end of the day to actually enjoy your evening, the principle is the same. A spine that's well-maintained and a nervous system that's running without interference make every one of those things easier. A spine that's breaking down quietly makes every one of them harder, often in ways you've stopped noticing because you've accepted the harder version as normal.

That acceptance is worth examining. How many things have you quietly written off as "just how I am now"? The afternoon energy crash. The stiffness that takes twenty minutes to clear in the morning. The tension headaches that show up after long meetings. The brain fog that makes the second half of your workday less sharp than the first. These aren't inevitable features of adult life. They are signals. And many of them trace back to a nervous system that's working harder than it should because the spine it depends on isn't giving it what it needs.

The performance case for spinal health isn't separate from the pain case. They are the same case at different points on the same scale. Pain is what happens when dysfunction has been building long enough to cross a threshold the nervous system can no longer ignore. Performance decline is what happens in the years before that threshold gets crossed. Addressing the spine before pain shows up doesn't just prevent the pain. It recovers the performance that was quietly slipping away while the degeneration was building in silence.

The Energy Connection — How Spinal Health Affects How You Feel All Day

Fatigue is one of the most common complaints that adults bring to their doctors. And one of the most common responses they get is a blood panel that comes back normal, followed by a recommendation to sleep more, stress less, and exercise more. The advice isn't wrong. But it's incomplete, because it misses one of the most consistent and least discussed drivers of chronic fatigue in otherwise healthy adults: a nervous system that's burning extra fuel to compensate for spinal dysfunction.

Here is the mechanism. When spinal joints are restricted and subluxations are present, the nervous system receives altered mechanical signals from those areas continuously. As previously described, the brain interprets these altered signals as a form of low-grade physical stress and responds by keeping the sympathetic nervous system partially activated. That sustained sympathetic tone doesn't feel like stress in the dramatic sense. It doesn't feel like anything specific at all. It just runs in the background, quietly consuming the neurological and metabolic resources that your body would otherwise be directing toward clarity, vitality, and recovery.

The analogy that makes this click for most people is a computer with too many background programs running. The processor isn't dedicated to what you're actively doing. It is splitting its resources between the task on the screen and a dozen processes running invisibly behind it. The computer slows down. Tasks take longer. The battery drains faster. You don't see the background programs. You just experience the sluggishness. A nervous system managing chronic spinal interference works exactly the same way. Your brain and body are capable of more, but the available resources are being partially consumed by a problem that's running in the background and never fully resolves.

People who start consistent chiropractic care frequently report one of the first noticeable changes is an increase in energy. Not after months of care. Often within the first few weeks. They sleep the same hours. Their diet hasn't changed. Their exercise habits are the same. But something shifted, and they feel more alert, more present, and less like they're pushing through the day. The explanation isn't mysterious. The nervous system is finally running with less interference. The background drain has been reduced. The resources that were being consumed compensating for spinal dysfunction are now available for the things that actually matter.

Consider a hypothetical scenario. Picture a 46-year-old financial analyst named David. He has been managing a low-grade fatigue for about three years. He sleeps seven hours a night, exercises twice a week, and eats reasonably well. His doctor has run his bloodwork twice and found nothing significant. He has been attributing the fatigue to the demands of his job and assuming it's just what his mid-forties feel like. He starts chiropractic care for an unrelated complaint, mild neck stiffness after a long flight. Three weeks into care, he notices that his afternoon energy crash has become less severe. By week six, it's largely gone. He's not doing anything else differently. The only change is that the cervical and upper thoracic subluxations that had been driving low-grade sympathetic activation in his nervous system for years are being progressively addressed. His nervous system is spending less energy compensating and more energy performing. This is a hypothetical example, but it reflects a pattern that chiropractors observe regularly in clinical practice.

The energy-spine connection also runs through sleep quality, which the next section covers in depth. But the daytime component is worth understanding on its own terms because it changes how you interpret the fatigue you're carrying. If you've been tired in a way that sleep doesn't fully fix, and your bloodwork is normal, and you've tried the standard recommendations without lasting results, the question worth asking is whether your nervous system has been running under interference that nobody has ever assessed. The answer to that question starts with a proper spinal evaluation, not another blood panel.

There is also a direct relationship between spinal health and the efficiency of the body's energy-producing systems. The nerves that regulate mitochondrial function, adrenal output, and thyroid activity all travel through or near the spinal column. When those pathways are operating without compression or irritation, the systems they serve can regulate themselves accurately. When those pathways are compromised, the regulation becomes less precise. The body's energy production becomes less efficient, not dramatically, but consistently, in a way that compounds over time into the kind of persistent, low-level fatigue that most people have stopped questioning because it's been there so long it feels like their baseline.

Your baseline isn't fixed. It is a reflection of the current state of your nervous system. Change the state of the nervous system by removing the interference that's been degrading it, and the baseline changes too. That is not a promise of boundless energy or a cure for every cause of fatigue. It is a straightforward description of what happens when a system that's been running below its capacity finally gets the conditions it needs to run properly.

Sleep, Recovery, and Spinal Health — The Overlooked Triangle

Sleep is when your body does its most important work. Not rest, exactly, though rest is part of it. The deep stages of sleep are when growth hormone is released, and tissue repair happens. When the brain clears metabolic waste through the glymphatic system. When the immune system consolidates its defenses. When the nervous system processes the day's sensory input and reorganizes its connections. When the emotional brain resets its calibration. None of that happens fully in light sleep. It happens in deep, restorative sleep. And getting into that deep sleep consistently requires one thing above almost everything else: a nervous system that's out of sympathetic overdrive.

A nervous system stuck in even low-grade sympathetic activation doesn't settle into deep sleep easily. It stays in a state of low-level alertness, monitoring for threats that aren't actually there, keeping the brain from fully releasing into the slow-wave and REM stages where the real restoration happens. People in this state often spend enough hours in bed but wake up feeling like they didn't sleep. They cycle through light sleep without ever dropping into the deeper stages long enough for the repair work to complete. They describe their sleep as "not refreshing" or say they "don't feel rested no matter how much they sleep." These are not just descriptions of tiredness. They are descriptions of a nervous system that couldn't fully switch off.

Spinal dysfunction contributes to this in two specific ways. The first is the mechanical stress signal pathway described in the previous section, where restricted spinal joints generate continuous altered input that keeps the sympathetic system partially activated. The second is more direct. Physical discomfort from spinal dysfunction, even discomfort that's too mild to register as pain during waking hours, becomes more noticeable when the body is still and trying to relax. The low-grade tension in the muscles around a restricted spinal segment, the subtle ache of a compressed nerve root, the discomfort of a disc that's loaded asymmetrically, these sensations that the busy, distracted waking mind easily overrides become more prominent when there's nothing else competing for the nervous system's attention. They create the kind of restlessness and light sleeping that people describe as "I just can't get comfortable" or "I keep waking up and I don't know why."

Many people who have struggled with poor sleep quality for years and tried every standard recommendation, sleep hygiene, limiting screens before bed, magnesium supplements, melatonin, white noise machines, have never had their spine assessed as a contributing factor. They have addressed the behavioral and environmental aspects of sleep without ever addressing the physical driver that's keeping the nervous system from settling. When that driver gets addressed through consistent spinal care, the sleep improvements that follow are often among the most dramatic and most quickly noticed changes people report. Not because chiropractic is a sleep treatment, but because removing the source of sympathetic activation allows the nervous system to do what it was already trying to do: settle down, switch gears, and let the body repair itself.

Recovery from physical activity is the other side of this triangle. Whether you're recovering from a workout, a physically demanding workday, or the general wear of being an active person, the quality of your recovery depends on how completely your nervous system can shift into parasympathetic mode during rest periods. The same spinal dysfunction that disrupts sleep disrupts recovery. Muscles that should be relaxing between training sessions stay slightly more contracted than they should. Inflammatory processes that should be resolving stay slightly more active. The tissues that should be rebuilding between sessions rebuild more slowly. Over time, this incomplete recovery compounds. Training adaptations come more slowly. Soreness lingers longer. Injury risk creeps up. The person who's doing everything right in their training but sleeping poorly and recovering slowly often has a nervous system problem, not a training problem.

The specific actions that address the sleep-spine connection are worth being concrete about. First, if you've been dealing with poor sleep quality that hasn't responded to standard sleep hygiene approaches, add a spinal assessment to your list of things to investigate. Ask your chiropractor specifically about the state of your upper cervical spine and whether any subluxations there could be reducing vagal tone and contributing to sympathetic dominance at night. This is a specific, answerable clinical question that gives you real information rather than guesswork.

Second, the evening spinal mobility sequence described previously, specifically the supine spinal twist and legs-up-the-wall position, is not just a movement practice. It is a deliberate parasympathetic activation protocol done at the time of day when shifting the nervous system toward recovery mode matters most. If you haven't incorporated it yet, start tonight. Five minutes before bed, on the floor next to your bed. The combination of gentle spinal decompression and the breathing that naturally deepens in these positions creates a measurable shift in autonomic tone that makes the transition into deep sleep significantly easier.

Third, sleeping position directly affects spinal mechanics during the hours when the body is trying to repair itself. The specifics described earlier bear repeating here in the context of sleep quality. Side-lying with a supportive pillow that keeps the cervical spine neutral and a pillow between the knees to keep the lumbar spine neutral is the position that minimizes mechanical stress on the spine during sleep. This isn't just about comfort. It is about reducing the physical input that can keep the nervous system from fully settling. A spine that's mechanically loaded during sleep is a spine whose surrounding muscles and nerve pathways are being stimulated during the hours when the body most needs to be free from that stimulation.

Mental Clarity, Mood, and the Spine — The Brain-Body Performance Loop

If you've read through the previous chapters, you already understand that the spine and the nervous system are inseparable. But most people still think of that connection primarily in physical terms. The spine affects how your back feels. It affects how you move. Maybe it affects your energy. What surprises people is how directly spinal health affects the brain itself, not just as a downstream effect of better sleep or lower stress, but as a direct, mechanistic influence on cognitive performance, mood, and emotional regulation.

Recall the concept of the brain-body loop described earlier, the continuous two-way conversation between the spine and the brain where the quality of sensory input traveling upward directly influences the quality of the brain's output traveling downward. That conversation is worth revisiting here specifically in the context of mental performance because the implications go significantly beyond what most people associate with back care.

The prefrontal cortex is the area of the brain responsible for the functions that define high-level human performance. Focus. Decision-making. Impulse control. Working memory. Creative problem-solving. Emotional regulation. The capacity to hold multiple pieces of information in mind simultaneously and reason through complex situations. These are the cognitive functions that determine how well you perform at work, how effectively you manage stress, how clearly you think under pressure, and how well you regulate your emotional responses to the inevitable challenges of daily life. And the prefrontal cortex is exquisitely sensitive to the quality of sensory input it receives from the body.

When spinal joints are healthy and moving through their full range, the mechanoreceptors in those joints generate a rich, varied stream of sensory input that travels up through the spinal cord to the brain. This input stimulates the cerebellum, which then activates the prefrontal cortex. The brain stays alert, calibrated, and operating at a high level. When spinal joints are restricted and that sensory stream drops, the stimulation to the prefrontal cortex decreases. The brain becomes less sharp. Focus becomes harder to maintain. Decision-making takes more effort. Emotional regulation becomes less reliable. These changes are subtle enough that most people don't connect them to their spine, but the neurological mechanism is direct and well-documented.

As mentioned, and described earlier, a study published in the Journal of Neural Plasticity found that spinal manipulation produced measurable changes in prefrontal cortex activity and improved sensorimotor processing in ways that persisted beyond the immediate post-adjustment period. Further, research measuring reaction time and cognitive accuracy before and after adjustments has consistently found improvements in both. These aren't the kinds of results you'd expect from a treatment that only affects the back. They are the results of a treatment that changes the quality of the brain's input, and therefore the quality of its output.

Mood is connected to this through several pathways. The most direct is the autonomic nervous system balance that spinal health influences. As we defined and discussed previously, chronic sympathetic dominance driven by spinal dysfunction keeps the brain in a state of low-grade threat response. The emotional brain, specifically the amygdala, stays more reactive than it should. Small stressors trigger larger responses. The emotional regulation capacity of the prefrontal cortex gets partially overridden by the threat-detection activity of the limbic system. People in this state describe feeling more irritable than their circumstances warrant, more anxious without a clear reason, more emotionally reactive in ways that feel out of character. They often attribute it to stress, which is partly right, but the physical driver of the nervous system imbalance is also contributing in a way that stress management alone can't fully address.

When spinal care shifts the nervous system back toward parasympathetic balance, the emotional brain recalibrates. The amygdala becomes less reactive. The prefrontal cortex regains more of its regulatory influence over emotional responses. People report feeling calmer, more even keeled, and more able to respond thoughtfully to situations that previously triggered disproportionate reactions. This isn't a psychological effect of feeling better about their health. It is a neurological effect of a nervous system that's no longer being kept in low-grade emergency mode by the physical input from a dysfunctional spine.

The serotonin connection adds another layer. Serotonin, which is the neurotransmitter most associated with mood stability, wellbeing, and emotional resilience, is produced primarily in the gut. The gut-brain axis, which is the bidirectional communication pathway between the enteric nervous system in the gut and the central nervous system in the brain, is regulated significantly by the vagus nerve. As previous chapters have established, vagal tone is directly influenced by cervical spine health. A cervical spine with good alignment and full mobility supports healthy vagal tone. Healthy vagal tone supports efficient gut-brain communication. Efficient gut-brain communication supports more stable serotonin production and signaling. The pathway from cervical spine health to mood stability runs through the vagus nerve and the gut, and it's more direct than most people would ever guess.

None of this means that spinal care is a treatment for depression or anxiety. It isn't and presenting it that way would be misleading. But it does mean that for people who are experiencing mood instability, difficulty concentrating, emotional reactivity, or a persistent mental fog that doesn't fully respond to the standard interventions, the spine and nervous system deserve to be part of the investigation. The brain doesn't operate in isolation from the body. It operates in constant, dynamic conversation with it. The quality of that conversation depends heavily on the health of the spine that carries it.

The practical implication of all this is straightforward. If you want to think more clearly, regulate your emotions more effectively, maintain sharper focus under pressure, and feel more mentally resilient in the face of daily demands, spinal health is a legitimate and underutilized tool for getting there. Not the only tool. But one that works through a direct, well-documented neurological mechanism that most people have never been told about. The spine isn't just the structure that holds you upright. It's a major sensory organ that feeds the brain the input it needs to perform at its best. Treat it accordingly, and the brain responds accordingly.

Your Quick-Start Guide

Everything in this chapter points toward a single, important reframe. Chiropractic care and spinal health aren't things you pursue when you're broken. They are things you maintain because you want to perform at your best, feel genuinely energized, sleep deeply, and think clearly. The spine is the gateway to the nervous system, and the nervous system is the gateway to every aspect of how you function, physically, mentally, and emotionally. Keeping that gateway clear isn't crisis management. It is intelligent, proactive investment in the quality of your daily life.

The entropy that this book has been describing from the first chapter doesn't stop working just because you're not in pain. It keeps chipping away, quietly, and consistently, at the structural and neurological foundations of your performance and vitality. The people who age well, who stay sharp and energetic and physically capable well into their later decades, aren't the ones who got lucky. They are the ones who decided early enough that maintenance was worth doing before breakdown made it unavoidable.

Here is a specific, numbered sequence to act on starting this week.

Step one: reframe your next chiropractic appointment, or your first one if you haven't started yet, as a performance assessment rather than a pain consultation. Go in with performance goals, not just symptom complaints. Tell your chiropractor what you want to be able to do, not just what hurts. Better sleep. Sharper thinking in the afternoon. More sustained energy. Faster recovery from workouts. These are legitimate clinical goals, and a good chiropractor will build your care plan around them.

Step two: starting today, track four specific metrics every evening for the next four weeks. Write them in a notebook, not a phone app, because the physical act of writing makes you more likely to notice and remember what you're recording. The four metrics are: energy level at 3 p.m. on a scale of one to ten, sleep quality the previous night on a scale of one to ten, mental sharpness and focus during your most demanding work period on a scale of one to ten, and overall physical ease of movement on a scale of one to ten. Four numbers, thirty seconds, every evening. After four weeks of consistent chiropractic care, compare your averages to your starting point. The data you collect will be more convincing than anything written in this chapter, because it will be your own body's response, measured in your own terms.

Step three: identify one person in your life who thinks chiropractic is only for people with back pain and share the energy, sleep, and brain-body performance concepts from this chapter with them. Not as a pitch. Just as information they probably haven't encountered before. The person who's been struggling with afternoon fatigue for two years and never connected it to their spine. The colleague who mentions they can't focus in the afternoons and assumes it's just the post-lunch slump. The family member who sleeps eight hours and still wakes up tired. The performance case for spinal health is genuinely surprising to most people the first time they hear it, because nobody told them the spine had anything to do with energy, sleep, or mental clarity. Now you know differently. Pass it along.

Step four: commit to a wellness care schedule with your chiropractor rather than stopping care when your symptoms resolve. Ask your chiropractor what maintenance frequency makes sense for your age, activity level, and spinal findings. For most adults, once or twice a month is the range that keeps the spine moving well, catches new restrictions before they compound, and maintains the nervous system function that the performance benefits in this chapter depend on. Wellness care isn't a commitment to being a patient forever. It is a commitment to treating your spine the way you treat your teeth, with regular maintenance that prevents the breakdown rather than waiting for the breakdown to force your hand.

The best version of your health isn't behind you. It is built in the choices you make from this point forward, one adjustment, one movement break, one good night of sleep, one clear-headed afternoon at a time.

Return to Work, Return to Play, Return to Function — The Recovery Roadmap

✦✦✦

The Three Milestones of Recovery — and Why They Matter in That Order

Recovery isn't a single moment. It is not the day the pain stops or the morning you wake up and notice the stiffness is gone. Recovery is a progression and understanding that progression changes everything about how you approach it, how long you stick with it, and how far you ultimately go.

There are three milestones that define a complete recovery from spinal dysfunction or injury. The first is returning to work, meaning you can handle the basic demands of daily life without pain getting in the way. The second is returning to play, meaning you can get back to the physical activities that make your life feel like yours. The third is returning to full function, meaning your spine and nervous system are operating at their best and you're not just surviving your days but genuinely thriving through them. Each milestone is distinct. Each one requires a different focus. And each one builds directly on the one before it.

"Return to work. Return to play. Return to function."

—Dr. Steven Roffers, DC

The order matters more than most people realize.

Skipping ahead is one of the most common and most costly mistakes people make during recovery. Someone feels well enough to jog again after two weeks of care, so they go out and run five miles. Someone's neck pain settles enough that they feel ready to return to their weekly tennis match, so they play a full set. Two days later, they're back where they started, sometimes worse. The problem isn't that they moved too soon. The problem is that they moved to the wrong level too soon before the foundation for that level had been built. Each milestone requires a specific level of structural stability, muscular support, and neurological readiness. Trying to skip to milestone two before milestone one is solid is like building the second floor of a house before the first floor walls are fully set. The structure can't hold the load.

Think about a hypothetical scenario. Picture a 47-year-old warehouse supervisor named Kevin. He's been dealing with a significant lumbar disc problem for about four months. He has been through the early phase of chiropractic care, and his pain has dropped from a seven out of ten to a two. He feels dramatically better. His chiropractor has been clear that he's still in the corrective phase of care and that his deep stabilizers are still being rebuilt, but Kevin feels good enough that he decides to go back to his weekend recreational soccer league. The first game goes fine. The second game, he takes an awkward step trying to change direction and feels a sharp pull in his lower back. He is now back up to a six out of ten in pain and has set his recovery back by several weeks. Kevin didn't fail at recovery. He just tried to run before he could walk, and the spine told him so. This is a hypothetical example, but it's one that chiropractors see play out regularly in clinical practice.

The three-milestone framework gives you a map. It tells you where you are, what the current phase requires, and what the next phase looks like so you can move toward it deliberately rather than impulsively. It replaces the guesswork of "am I ready for this?" with a clear set of criteria that you and your chiropractor can evaluate together. And it reframes recovery not as a straight line from pain to no pain, but as a structured progression from basic function to full capacity, with specific goals and specific strategies at each stage.

Every section that follows covers one of these milestones in detail, including what it looks like, what care and rehabilitation strategies are most effective at that stage, and exactly how to know when you're ready to move forward. The final section covers how chiropractic care and rehabilitation work together throughout the entire process. By the time you finish this chapter, you'll have a complete, specific picture of what a genuine recovery looks like from start to finish.

Return to Work — Getting Your Body Back to the Demands of Daily Life

The first milestone of recovery is deceptively simple. It sounds like a low bar. Get back to work. Handle the basics. Move through your day without the pain running the show. But for someone who's been significantly limited by spinal dysfunction, this milestone represents a genuine achievement, and reaching it correctly is what makes everything that follows possible.

Return to work doesn't just mean your job. It means the full range of basic daily demands. Driving without pain. Sitting through a meeting. Walking the grocery store. Getting in and out of the car without bracing. Picking up something light from the floor. Sleeping through the night without being woken by discomfort. These are the activities that define functional daily life, and when spinal dysfunction has taken them away, getting them back is the first and most urgent goal of recovery.

The primary focus at this stage is reducing the acute dysfunction that's limiting basic movement. This means addressing the active subluxations and nerve irritation that are producing the most significant symptoms, reducing the protective muscle guarding around affected spinal segments, and beginning to restore the range of motion that's been lost. Chiropractic adjustments during this phase are typically more frequent, often two to three times per week, because the spine needs consistent input to begin shifting out of the restricted, inflamed state it's been locked into. Each adjustment builds on the previous one. The nervous system needs repetition to start recalibrating, and the joints need repeated, correct movement to begin releasing the protective tension that's been holding them in place.

Pain management during this phase is real and important, but it should never be the only goal. The mistake most people make at this stage is treating pain relief as the finish line. Pain drops to a manageable level, they feel like the problem is solved, and they stop care. As this book has covered from the beginning, pain is a late signal. It was the last thing to arrive, and it's the first thing to leave, long before the underlying structural and neurological correction has been completed. Stopping care when the pain improves is like stopping a course of antibiotics after three days because you feel better. The symptom has responded, but the underlying problem hasn't been resolved.

Rehabilitation at the return-to-work stage is gentle and targeted. The goal isn't to build strength yet. The goal is to restore basic movement patterns that pain and protective guarding have disrupted. This means reactivating muscles that have been inhibited by the dysfunction and beginning to move the spine through its pain-free range without loading it beyond what it can currently handle. Walking is one of the most appropriate and most underused rehabilitation tools at this stage. As we previously established, walking loads the lumbar discs rhythmically through the imbibition cycle, activates the gluteal muscles that support the lumbar spine, and drives thoracic rotation that keeps the mid-back mobile. Start with whatever distance and duration is comfortable and pain-free. Ten minutes is enough to start. The consistency matters far more than the distance at this point.

The specific criteria for knowing you've completed the return-to-work milestone are these. You can sit for at least thirty minutes without significant pain increase. You can walk for at least fifteen to twenty minutes at a comfortable pace without symptoms worsening. You can perform your basic daily tasks, including your job's primary physical demands, without needing to stop or significantly modify what you're doing because of pain. Your pain level at rest is consistently at a two out of ten or below. And your chiropractor's assessment confirms that the acute nerve irritation has settled and the affected spinal segments are beginning to move more freely between appointments. All five of these criteria need to be met, not just one or two. When they are, you're ready to move to the next phase.

Two things to protect during the return-to-work phase that most people don't think about carefully enough. First, your sleep position. The structural changes that happen during the day need the nighttime hours to begin consolidating. A sleeping position that mechanically stresses the recovering spinal segments undoes some of what the day's care has accomplished. Side-lying with a neutral cervical pillow and a pillow between the knees for lumbar and hip alignment is the position that minimizes mechanical load during sleep and gives the recovering tissues the best environment for repair. Second, your sitting posture during the workday. If you sit for your job, the lumbar support and monitor height corrections we previously defined and discussed aren't optional during recovery. They are essential. Spending eight hours a day in a posture that recreates the mechanical loading that caused the problem in the first place means your adjustments are fighting against your daily environment rather than being supported by it.

Return to Play — Getting Back to the Activities That Make Life Worth Living

The second milestone is the one that matters most emotionally. Return to work is about function. Return to play is about identity. The activity you love, whether that's golf, hiking, swimming, cycling, playing with your grandchildren, training for a race, or simply being able to walk your dog for an hour without paying for it the next day, represents a part of who you are. When spinal dysfunction takes that away, it doesn't just cause physical limitation. It takes something from your quality of life that pain management alone can't restore.

Getting back to play requires a deliberate, structured approach. Not because it's inherently dangerous, but because the activities that fall into this category make demands on the spine that are significantly higher than the demands of basic daily life. A golf swing loads the lumbar spine with rotational forces that far exceed what sitting at a desk does. Hiking on uneven terrain challenges the proprioceptive system and the deep stabilizers in ways that walking on flat ground doesn't. Picking up a grandchild combines a loaded forward bend with a dynamic lift, which is one of the higher-demand movement patterns for the lumbar spine. These activities are achievable. But they require a foundation that has to be built deliberately during the transition from milestone one to milestone two.

The central focus of the return-to-play phase is building the structural resilience and neuromuscular control that higher-demand activities require. This is where rehabilitation becomes more specific and more progressive. The deep stabilizer activation work that began in the return-to-work phase gets more challenging. The movement pattern retraining described earlier becomes more sport-specific or activity-specific. The progressive loading that rebuilds spinal strength and resilience moves from basic bodyweight exercises to more demanding patterns that mirror the actual demands of the activities you're returning to.

Chiropractic care during the return-to-play phase typically drops to once or twice a week. The acute dysfunction has been addressed. The focus now is on ensuring that the spinal segments that were most affected are moving freely and staying in correct alignment as the mechanical demands being placed on the spine increase. Regular adjustments at this stage serve two purposes. They catch any new restrictions that develop as training loads increase before those restrictions have time to compound. And they maintain the nervous system function that proprioception, coordination, and movement efficiency depend on. The athlete who gets adjusted regularly during a return-to-sport progression consistently shows better movement quality, faster skill reacquisition, and lower re-injury rates than the athlete who relies on rehabilitation exercises alone. The combination is what produces the best outcomes.

The progression back to higher-demand activities needs to be gradual and specific. Here is a concrete framework for how to approach it. Start at twenty-five percent of your pre-injury activity level. If you used to hike five miles, start with one and a quarter. If you used to play eighteen holes of golf, start with four or five holes. If you used to run thirty minutes, start with seven or eight. Do this reduced level for one week without any significant symptom increase. If you feel fine at the end of that week, meaning your pain hasn't increased beyond a one out of ten above your current baseline during or after the activity, increase to fifty percent the following week. Continue this twenty-five percent weekly progression until you're back at your full pre-injury level. If at any point during this progression your symptoms increase beyond a one out of ten above baseline during the activity, or if they're still elevated twenty-four hours after the activity, stop at that level for an additional week before attempting to progress again. This isn't timid caution. It is the specific protocol that prevents the re-injury cycle that sets so many people back.

There is a psychological dimension to the return-to-play phase that deserves honest acknowledgment. After a significant period of pain and limitation, many people develop a fear-avoidance pattern where they start to anticipate pain before it arrives and restrict their movement preemptively. This is a completely understandable response to months of being taught by their own body that certain movements hurt. But it becomes a barrier to recovery if it's not addressed, because the nervous system learns from what you do, and consistently avoiding movements that are actually safe to perform reinforces the neural pathways that associate those movements with threat. If you notice that you're avoiding activities that your chiropractor and rehabilitation provider have cleared you to attempt, bring that up explicitly. A graduated exposure approach, where you systematically practice the avoided movements in a controlled, supported environment, directly addresses this pattern and is an important part of a complete return-to-play plan.

The criteria for completing the return-to-play milestone are these. You can perform your chosen activity at your pre-injury level without symptoms exceeding a one out of ten above your resting baseline during or after the activity. Your spinal segments are moving freely and holding their correction between adjustments. Your deep stabilizers are activating reliably during the activity, which your chiropractor or rehabilitation provider can assess through functional movement testing. And you feel confident, not fearful, in your body's ability to handle the demands of the activity. Confidence that's based on demonstrated capacity, not wishful thinking. When all of these are true, you're ready for the final milestone.

Return to Function — Living at Full Capacity Without Limits

The third milestone is where most people never arrive, not because it's unachievable, but because they stopped at milestone one or two and called it done. They got out of pain. They got back to their activities. They felt good enough. And "good enough" quietly became the new ceiling.

Return to full function is something different. It is not just the absence of pain or the return to previous activities. It's a spine and nervous system that are operating at their genuine best, with the structural integrity, muscular support, and neurological clarity that allow you to move through life without limitation, without fear of breakdown, and without the quiet background drain that compromised spinal health creates in your energy, sleep, and mental performance. It is what the previous chapter described as the performance case for spinal health, applied as the endpoint of a complete recovery rather than as a separate goal for athletes and high performers.

Full function looks different for different people, and it's important to define it specifically for yourself rather than using a generic standard. For a 32-year-old runner, full function might mean training for and completing a half marathon without any spinal symptoms and with improved running economy compared to pre-injury. For a 58-year-old office worker, it might mean sitting through a full workday without any neck or lower back symptoms, sleeping through the night without discomfort, and hiking on weekends without the next-day stiffness that used to follow. For a 73-year-old grandparent, it means being able to pick up grandchildren, gardening for an hour, and walking the dog daily without any of those activities producing the symptoms that limited them before. The specific picture is personal. But the principle is universal: Full function means doing everything you want to do, at the level you want to do it, without your spine or nervous system being the limiting factor.

Reaching full function requires addressing several elements that the earlier phases of recovery laid the groundwork for but didn't fully complete. The first is comprehensive spinal strength. The deep stabilizers that were reactivated and trained during the return-to-work and return-to-play phases need to be developed to a level of endurance and load capacity that can handle the full range of demands that daily life and chosen activities place on them. This means progressive resistance training that loads the spine in its corrected alignment and through its full range of motion. Deadlifts, squats, carries, and rows done with proper form and progressively increasing load are among the most effective tools for building this strength. The specific exercises and loading progression should be developed in collaboration with your chiropractor and rehabilitation provider based on your spinal findings and your functional goals.

The second element is neurological optimization. As previously covered, a healthy, mobile spine feeds the brain rich sensory input that keeps motor control precise, proprioception accurate, and cognitive function sharp. At the full function milestone, the goal is to ensure that the spine is providing this input at its maximum quality. This means regular chiropractic maintenance adjustments to keep all spinal segments moving freely, combined with movement practices that challenge the proprioceptive system progressively. Balance training, coordination drills, and complex movement patterns that require the spine to adapt dynamically all contribute to this neurological optimization. The person who has reached full function isn't just pain-free. They're moving better, thinking more clearly, and recovering from physical demands faster than they were before the injury that started the recovery process.

The third element is the maintenance system that prevents entropy from quietly reclaiming the ground you've worked to recover. This is the most critical and most often neglected part of the full function milestone. The entropy that we described earlier doesn't stop working because you've completed a recovery program. It keeps working, every day, on every unattended structure. The gains made through recovery are real and significant, but they're not permanent by default. They require ongoing maintenance to hold. Regular spinal adjustments, consistent daily movement, the posture habits we discussed, the movement breaks we described, the parasympathetic practices we defined and described: these aren't things you do during recovery and then stop. They're the ongoing inputs that keep the system running at the level you've worked to achieve.

The specific maintenance schedule that supports full function for most adults is monthly spinal adjustments, daily spinal mobility work of ten to fifteen minutes, three to four days per week of progressive strength training that includes spinal loading, daily walking of at least twenty to thirty minutes, and the workday movement breaks every forty-five minutes that we described previously. This is not a demanding regimen. It is a sustainable daily practice that, done consistently, keeps the entropy at bay and preserves the function you've built. Think of it as the maintenance schedule for the most important structure you own.

How do you know you've reached full function? The criteria are specific. Your pain is consistently at zero or near zero at rest and during all chosen activities. Your spinal segments are moving freely throughout their full range and holding their correction between monthly maintenance adjustments. Your deep stabilizers are strong enough to handle your highest-demand activities without fatigue or breakdown. Your energy, sleep quality, and mental clarity are at a level that you'd describe as genuinely good, not just acceptable. And you're not managing your spine, you're maintaining it, with a proactive daily practice rather than a reactive response to symptoms. When all of these are true, you've completed the recovery roadmap. You are not a patient anymore. You are a person who takes care of their spine the way it deserves to be taken care of.

The Role of Rehabilitation and Physical Therapy in the Recovery Process

Chiropractic adjustments and rehabilitation are not competing approaches. They are two halves of the same complete solution and understanding how they work together changes how you think about your care plan at every stage of recovery.

Here is the simplest way to understand the distinction. A chiropractic adjustment restores motion to a restricted joint, reduces nerve interference, and resets the neurological patterns around that joint. It opens the door. Rehabilitation builds the muscular support, movement patterns, and neuromuscular control that keep the door open. Without the adjustment, rehabilitation is being done through a spine that still has mechanical restrictions limiting its range and distorting its movement patterns.

Without rehabilitation, the adjustments don't hold as well because the muscles and ligaments that surround the corrected segments haven't been retrained to support the corrected position under load. The two approaches need each other to produce results that last.

Physical therapy contributes specific tools that complement the chiropractic component of care at every phase of recovery. Soft tissue work, including myofascial release and trigger point therapy, addresses the chronic muscle tension and fascial restrictions that develop around subluxated areas and that limit the range of motion available for both adjustments and rehabilitation exercises. Manual therapy techniques that restore mobility to joints adjacent to the primary area of dysfunction reduce the compensatory patterns that develop when one spinal region has been restricted for a long time. Therapeutic modalities like electrical stimulation and ultrasound can reduce acute inflammation and muscle spasm in ways that make the spine more receptive to adjustments and more capable of performing rehabilitation exercises correctly.

The exercise prescription component of physical therapy is where the most specific and most individualized work happens. A good rehabilitation program isn't a generic set of back exercises. It is a carefully sequenced progression that starts with what the spine can currently do without pain or compensatory movement and systematically advances toward what the spine needs to be able to do to meet the person's functional goals. That progression moves through the four categories previously described: mobility restoration, deep stabilizer activation, movement pattern retraining, and progressive loading. The sequencing matters. Trying to load a spine that hasn't had its movement patterns corrected first reinforces the dysfunctional patterns. Trying to retrain movement patterns before the deep stabilizers have been activated means the movement will be driven by the outer muscles that are already overworked rather than the inner muscles that provide the precise, moment-to-moment stability the spine needs.

Communication between your chiropractor and your rehabilitation provider is not optional if you want the best possible outcomes. It is essential. The chiropractor's assessment tells the rehabilitation provider which segments are restricted, which nerve pathways are compromised, and which movement patterns are being distorted by the spinal dysfunction. The rehabilitation provider's assessment tells the chiropractor which muscles are inhibited, which movement compensations are present, and which exercises are producing the best neurological response. When these two professionals share information and coordinate their approach, the care plan they build together is more targeted, more efficient, and more effective than either could produce working independently. When you're choosing your care providers, ask specifically whether they communicate with each other about shared patients. If the answer is no, that's a significant gap in your care that's worth addressing.

The integration of chiropractic and rehabilitation also changes over the course of the recovery timeline in ways that are worth understanding. During the return-to-work phase, adjustments are more frequent and rehabilitation is gentle, focused on basic movement restoration. As you move into the return-to-play phase, adjustment frequency decreases and rehabilitation becomes more specific and more demanding, building the capacity for higher-level activities. At the full function phase, adjustments shift to monthly maintenance and rehabilitation transitions into a self-managed daily practice, with periodic check-ins with your rehabilitation provider to ensure the program is progressing appropriately and to address any new restrictions or compensations that develop.

"Chiropractors can play an important role in strengthening rehabilitation in health systems as they deliver interventions for rehabilitation for people with health conditions throughout the life course, and across the continuum of care."

—Katie de Luca, MChiro, PhD
Central Queensland University,
Brisbane, Australia

One of the most important things to understand about this integrated approach is that it addresses the root cause of the problem rather than just managing its symptoms. A person who receives only pain management, whether through medication, passive modalities, or rest, may feel better temporarily. But the mechanical dysfunction that caused the problem hasn't been corrected, the muscular support that should protect the spine hasn't been rebuilt, and the movement patterns that were loading the spine incorrectly haven't been retrained. The problem that produced the symptoms is still there, waiting to produce them again. A person who receives integrated chiropractic and rehabilitation care, done correctly and carried through to the full function milestone, has addressed all three of these layers. The spine is moving correctly. The muscles are supporting it correctly. The movement patterns are loading it correctly. That's a genuinely different outcome, and it's the difference between managing a recurring problem and actually solving it.

Putting It Into Practice

Recovery is a three-stage progression, and each stage has a specific purpose, specific criteria, and a specific set of strategies that make it work. Return to work restores basic daily function. Return to play restores the activities that make life meaningful. Return to full function builds a body that operates at its genuine best and maintains that level through consistent, proactive care. Skipping stages or stopping early produces incomplete results. Completing all three produces something genuinely different: a spine and nervous system that aren't just recovered but optimized.

The entropy that's been working on your body since the day you were born doesn't stop working because you've had a good month of care. It keeps going, quietly and consistently, the way it always has. The recovery roadmap in this chapter isn't just a path out of pain. It's a framework for building the kind of ongoing relationship with your spine that keeps entropy from winning back the ground you've worked to recover. That is the real goal. Not just getting better. Staying better and building from there.

Three specific actions to take starting this week.

First, identify which stage of recovery you're currently in and write down, on paper, what full function looks like for you specifically. Not a generic description. Your description. The activities you want to return to, the energy level you want to have, the physical demands you want to be able to meet without limitation. Make it concrete enough that you'd know without question whether you'd achieved it. This written picture becomes the target that every decision about your care is aimed at.

Second, bring that written picture to your next chiropractic appointment and ask your chiropractor to build a progression plan with you that has specific milestones, specific timelines, and specific criteria for moving from one stage to the next. Ask which rehabilitation exercises are most important for your current stage, what the adjustment frequency should be at each phase, and how you'll know when you're ready to progress. A care plan without specific milestones is a plan without a destination. Get the specifics in writing so you can track your progress against something concrete.

Third, commit to not stopping care when the pain stops. Make that commitment now, before the pain stops, because that's when the temptation to stop will be strongest. The pain stopping is not the finish line. It is the point at which the deeper, more important work of structural correction, muscular rebuilding, and neurological optimization begins. The people who reach full function are the ones who understood this before they got there and stayed the course because of it. Be one of those people.

Treatment From the Inside Out — Why the Body Heals Better Without Interference

✦✦✦

Inside-Out vs. Outside-In — Two Fundamentally Different Models of Health

There are two completely different ways to think about how the body gets better.

The first way is the one most of us grew up with. Something goes wrong. You feel it. You go to a doctor or a pharmacy. Something external is applied to the problem. A drug suppresses the symptom. An injection reduces the inflammation. A surgery removes or repairs the damaged structure. The body is treated as the problem, and the solution comes from outside it. This is the outside-in model of healthcare, and it's the dominant model in conventional medicine. It's also genuinely useful in the right situations. Nobody is arguing that a broken bone should be left to sort itself out or that a serious infection doesn't need antibiotics.

But there's a second model. And for a very large category of health problems, it's more powerful, more lasting, and more aligned with how the body actually works.

The inside-out model starts from a different premise entirely. Instead of asking "what can we apply from the outside to suppress this symptom," it asks "what is getting in the way of the body doing what it already knows how to do?" The goal isn't to override the body's processes. The goal is to remove whatever is interfering with them. Clear the path. Restore the conditions the body needs to self-regulate, self-heal, and self-organize. And then get out of the way.

Chiropractic care is built on this model. The spine is the protective housing for the nervous system, and the nervous system is the master controller of every healing, regulatory, and restorative process in the body. When the spine is misaligned, when joints are restricted, when nerve pathways are compressed, the body's ability to heal itself gets throttled. Not dramatically, at least not at first. But consistently, quietly, and cumulatively. The inside-out approach says: find the interference, remove it, and let the body do what it was designed to do.

This isn't anti-medicine. It is a recognition that medicine works best when it's used for what it's actually designed for, and that a huge portion of what people reach for conventional medicine to fix has an inside-out cause that outside-in tools can only manage, never resolve.

Think about what happens when you get a splinter in your finger. The right intervention is to remove the splinter. Your body handles the rest. The inflammation, the tissue repair, the healing of the skin, all of that is your innate intelligence doing its job the moment the interference is removed. Now imagine instead that you left the splinter in and just took anti-inflammatories every day to manage the swelling. The swelling would reduce. The pain would be more manageable. But the splinter would still be there, the inflammation would keep coming back, and the tissue would never fully heal because the cause of the problem was never addressed. That is not a dramatic example. That is exactly what happens when people manage spinal dysfunction with pain medication for years without ever addressing the mechanical interference driving it.

The inside-out model changes the question you ask about your health. Instead of "what can I take to make this feel better," the question becomes "what is preventing my body from fixing this on its own, and how do I remove it?" That is a more powerful question. It leads to more powerful answers. And it's the question that chiropractic care has been built around since D.D. Palmer asked it in 1895.

Understanding this distinction isn't just intellectually interesting. It changes every practical decision you make about your health. It changes which interventions you reach for first. It changes how you evaluate whether a treatment is actually working or just masking the problem. It changes your relationship with your own body, from passive recipient of external fixes to active participant in a healing process your body is already trying to complete. That shift in perspective is one of the most valuable things this chapter can give you, because it reframes every health decision you'll make from this point forward.

The entropy that this book has been describing from the first chapter is, at its core, a story about interference accumulating over time. Poor posture creates mechanical interference. Subluxations create neurological interference. Chronic stress creates autonomic interference. Sedentary behavior creates nutritional interference in the discs and joints. All of these forms of interference compound on each other, quietly degrading the body's ability to maintain itself. The inside-out model addresses entropy at its source by systematically removing the interference that's allowing it to win. That is not a metaphor. That is the mechanism.

When Outside-In Treatment Makes Sense — and When It Doesn't

Being honest about this matters. Outside-in treatment isn't the enemy. It has a real and important role in healthcare and dismissing it entirely would be both inaccurate and irresponsible.

There are situations where outside-in intervention is the right tool, the best tool, and sometimes the only tool. Acute trauma with structural damage needs surgical repair. A serious bacterial infection needs antibiotics. Severe, debilitating pain that's preventing a person from sleeping or functioning needs short-term management while the underlying cause is being addressed. A disc herniation that's producing progressive neurological deficits, meaning actual loss of strength or sensation in the limbs, may need surgical decompression if conservative care hasn't produced adequate improvement in a reasonable timeframe. These situations exist. They are real. And in those situations, outside-in medicine is exactly where you want to be.

The problem isn't that outside-in treatment exists. The problem is how broadly it gets applied to problems it wasn't designed to solve.

Consider a hypothetical scenario. Picture a 48-year-old project manager named Sarah. She has been dealing with chronic lower back pain for about three years. It started after a period of intense work stress, long hours at her desk, and a complete drop-off in physical activity. Her doctor prescribed a muscle relaxant and an anti-inflammatory, which helped for a while. When the pain came back, the doses were increased. When that stopped working as well, she was referred for a cortisone injection. The injection gave her about six weeks of relief. Then the pain returned. She's now being evaluated for a second injection and has been told that if that doesn't work, a surgical consultation might be appropriate. At no point in this three-year process has anyone assessed her spinal alignment, evaluated her for subluxations, analyzed her posture, or addressed the mechanical dysfunction that's been driving the inflammation that the injections keep temporarily suppressing. The outside-in tools she's been given are real and they work for what they're designed for. But they're being used to manage a problem that has an inside-out cause, and that mismatch is why she's still in pain three years later. This is a hypothetical example, but it reflects a pattern that is extraordinarily common in the management of chronic spinal pain.

The mismatch between an outside-in tool and an inside-out problem is one of the most expensive and most common mistakes in modern healthcare. It is expensive in the obvious financial sense, because managing a chronic problem with repeated interventions that don't address the root costs significantly more over time than addressing the root once. But it's also expensive in terms of function, quality of life, and the progressive structural deterioration that continues while the symptoms are being managed but the cause is being ignored. Every month that the mechanical interference driving a problem goes unaddressed is another month of entropy winning ground that becomes harder and harder to recover.

The distinction that matters most is this: is the treatment addressing the cause, or is it addressing the symptom? Outside-in treatments almost always address the symptom. That's useful when the symptom is severe enough to be dangerous or debilitating, and when addressing the cause requires time that the symptom won't allow. But it becomes a trap when symptom management becomes the permanent strategy rather than a temporary bridge to root-cause care.

Pain medication reduces pain. It doesn't restore spinal alignment. Anti-inflammatories reduce inflammation. They don't correct the mechanical stress that's generating the inflammation. Cortisone injections suppress the local inflammatory response. They don't address the subluxation or disc dysfunction that's triggering it. Muscle relaxants reduce muscle spasm. They don't release the joint restriction that the spasm is protecting. Each of these interventions has a legitimate short-term role. None of them, used alone and long-term, changes the underlying trajectory of a spine that's breaking down because of mechanical interference that hasn't been removed.

The smarter approach is to use outside-in interventions deliberately and temporarily, as tools that create a window of reduced pain and inflammation within which inside-out care can do its work. Take the anti-inflammatory to get the acute inflammation down enough that the spine can be assessed and adjusted. Use the pain medication short-term to get through the worst days while the underlying dysfunction is being addressed. Consider the injection if pain is severe enough that it's preventing you from participating in the rehabilitation that's going to make the lasting difference. But always know what the outside-in tool is doing and what it isn't doing. Always have an inside-out plan running alongside it. And always have a clear endpoint for the outside-in intervention rather than letting it become an indefinite management strategy for a problem that has a solvable root cause.

The practical question to ask yourself about any treatment you're currently using is straightforward. Is this addressing why my body is struggling, or is it managing what my body is experiencing because of why it's struggling? If the answer is the second one, the next question is: what is the root cause, and is anyone addressing it? If nobody is, that gap is the most important thing to close in your current health strategy.

Building a Health Strategy That Works With Your Body, Not Against It

Most people don't have a health strategy. They have a collection of reactions. Something hurts; they react. Something gets worse, they react more. The reactions might be intelligent and well-chosen, but they're still reactions. They are responses to problems that have already arrived rather than a proactive plan for keeping those problems from arriving in the first place.

A genuine health strategy is different. It is built around the inside-out model, it uses outside-in tools wisely when they're needed, and it defaults to root-cause care as the foundation rather than symptom management as the plan. Building that strategy doesn't require a medical degree. It requires understanding a few clear principles and making a handful of specific, consistent decisions.

The foundation of an inside-out health strategy is regular spinal care. Not reactive care that starts when something hurts and stops when the pain goes away. Maintenance care that keeps the spine moving properly, catches new restrictions before they compound, and keeps the nervous system running without the interference that quietly degrades everything from your energy and sleep to your immune function and cognitive performance. As we previously covered, this is the wellness care model. Monthly adjustments for most adults in good spinal health. More frequent care during periods of higher physical demand, increased stress, or when new dysfunction is being addressed. The frequency is calibrated to the individual, but the principle is consistent: regular maintenance beats crisis management every time, in both outcomes and cost.

Movement is the second pillar. Not exercise as an optional add-on, but daily, intentional movement as a biological requirement for spinal health. The morning mobility sequence, the workday movement breaks, the daily walk, the progressive strength training that rebuilds the muscular support around the spine, all of it working together to keep the discs nourished, the joints mobile, the deep stabilizers activated, and the proprioceptive input to the brain rich and accurate. The health strategy previously defined and described is what makes that framework a non-negotiable daily practice rather than something you do when you remember to.

Nutrition is the third pillar, specifically in its role in managing the systemic inflammation that accelerates spinal degeneration and makes the nervous system's job harder. The specific nutrition and diet changes we discussed previously apply here: replacing refined vegetable oils with olive oil, adding fatty fish twice a week or supplementing with two grams of combined EPA and DHA daily, and reducing added sugar below twenty-five grams per day. These aren't dramatic dietary overhauls. They're targeted reductions in the inflammatory load the body is operating under, and they directly support every other element of the inside-out strategy.

Sleep is the fourth pillar, and it's the one that ties everything else together. As we covered in detail earlier, deep restorative sleep is when the body does its most important repair work. A health strategy that doesn't protect sleep quality is a strategy with a significant leak. The specific actions are concrete: no bright screens in the ninety minutes before bed, a cool bedroom between 65 and 68 degrees Fahrenheit, a sleeping position that keeps the spine neutral, and the evening spinal decompression practice that shifts the nervous system toward parasympathetic recovery before sleep. These aren't complicated. They are consistent, and consistency is what makes them work.

Stress management is the fifth pillar, specifically through its effect on the sympathetic-parasympathetic balance that we described in detail previously. The five-minute diaphragmatic breathing practice every morning, the deliberate protection of parasympathetic recovery time, the daily walk that reduces cortisol and improves vagal tone, and the regular social connection that directly activates the parasympathetic system through the mechanisms Stephen Porges' polyvagal research identified. These practices don't eliminate stress. They prevent the nervous system from getting locked in the chronic sympathetic dominance that degrades spinal health, immune function, sleep quality, and cognitive performance simultaneously.

These five pillars work together as a system, and that's the key word. They are not five separate things you do for five separate reasons. They are five inputs into the same system, the spine and nervous system that controls everything else. When all five are in place, the system runs well. When any one of them is consistently missing, the others can partially compensate but can't fully replace what's absent. A person who gets adjusted regularly but sleeps poorly, moves little, and eats in a way that drives systemic inflammation is leaving most of the potential benefit of their chiropractic care unrealized. A person who eats well and exercises but never gets their spine assessed is maintaining everything around the central system while leaving the central system itself unattended. The strategy works because all five pillars are present and consistent, not because any one of them is perfect.

The most important shift in building this strategy is the shift from reactive to proactive. Reactive health management waits for the signal. Proactive health management doesn't need a signal because it's already maintaining the system. The reactive approach is more expensive, produces worse outcomes, and leaves the person feeling like a victim of their own body. The proactive approach costs less over time, produces dramatically better outcomes, and gives the person a sense of genuine agency over their health that most people have never experienced. That agency is one of the most significant benefits of understanding and applying the inside-out model, because it changes your relationship with your body from adversarial to collaborative.

Your body isn't working against you. It never has been. Every symptom you've experienced, every alarm your body has sounded, every signal you've tried to suppress with an outside-in intervention, was your body trying to communicate something that needed to be addressed. The inside-out model teaches you to listen to those communications and respond to their cause rather than silencing them and hoping the problem resolves on its own. That is a fundamentally different way of living in your body, and it's the approach that the research, the clinical outcomes, and the basic biology all point toward as the most effective long-term strategy for staying healthy, functional, and genuinely well.

What to Do With This

The inside-out model is not a philosophy. It is a practical framework for making better decisions about your health every single day. Understanding it is the starting point. Applying it is what actually changes things.

Here are three specific actions to take before you move on to the final chapter.

First, review your current health habits and identify which ones are treating symptoms and which ones are addressing root causes. Make two columns on a piece of paper. In the first column, list everything you currently do or take to manage symptoms: the ibuprofen for the headaches, the antacids for the reflux, the sleep aid for the insomnia, the muscle rub for the back tension. In the second column, list everything you currently do that addresses root causes: the chiropractic adjustments, the daily movement, the sleep position corrections, the anti-inflammatory nutritional changes. Look at the balance between the two columns honestly. If the first column is significantly longer than the second, you have a clear picture of where your strategy needs to shift. Pick one item from the first column and identify the specific root-cause intervention that could replace it over the next thirty days.

Second, have a specific conversation with your chiropractor at your next appointment about building a formal inside-out health strategy. Come in with the five pillars from this chapter written down. Ask your chiropractor to assess which pillars are currently in place and which have gaps. Ask for specific recommendations for each gap, not general advice. If movement is the gap, ask which specific exercises are most important for your spinal findings right now. If sleep is the gap, ask whether your cervical spine findings could be contributing to poor sleep quality and what the treatment plan for that looks like. If stress is the gap, ask which areas of your spine are most likely contributing to sympathetic activation and how the current care plan is addressing them. Specific questions produce specific answers, and specific answers are what allow you to build a strategy that actually fits your body rather than a generic plan that fits nobody in particular.

Third, reduce your reliance on over-the-counter pain management by one concrete step this month and replace it with a root-cause intervention. If you currently take ibuprofen three or four times a week for recurring back or neck pain, set a specific target of reducing that to once a week by replacing the other instances with the ten-minute morning mobility sequence, an additional walk, and ice or heat applied to the affected area. If you currently take something for headaches two or three times a week, book a cervical spine assessment this week to determine whether the headaches have a spinal component that's never been addressed. The goal isn't to eliminate pain management entirely or to suffer through pain unnecessarily. The goal is to make root-cause intervention the first response and outside-in management the backup, rather than the other way around. That single reversal in priority, applied consistently, changes the long-term trajectory of your spinal health more than any individual treatment decision could.

The body you're living in right now is the same body that has been trying to heal, regulate, and restore itself your entire life. It hasn't stopped trying. It just needs the interference removed. That's what the inside-out model gives it. That is what this entire book has been pointing toward. Remove the interference, support the system, and let the most sophisticated self-healing mechanism in the known universe do what it was built to do.

Your Anti-Entropy Plan — The Daily Blueprint for a Body That Lasts

✦✦✦

Everything in this book has been building toward this chapter.

The entropy that's been quietly working on your spine since your twenties. The nervous system that controls every function in your body and depends on a healthy spine to do its job. The subluxations that create interference you can't feel until the damage is already significant. The inside-out model that removes the cause rather than managing the symptom. All of it has been pointing toward one question: what do you actually do about it, every day, in a real life with real demands and limited time?

That is what this chapter answers.

Not in vague terms. Not with advice like "move more" or "reduce stress." With a specific, practical, daily blueprint that takes everything covered in the previous eleven chapters and turns it into a plan you can actually execute. A plan built around a system that actually works. A set of daily habits that are small enough to be sustainable but powerful enough to compound into real, lasting change. And a way to measure your progress that keeps you honest and motivated over the long haul.

The people who age well, who stay sharp and physically capable and genuinely energetic well into their later decades, don't do one thing perfectly. They do several things consistently. That consistency, applied over months and years, is what separates a body that holds up from one that quietly falls apart. The anti-entropy plan in this chapter is built around that principle. It is not a program you do for thirty days and then stop. It is a way of living in your body that you maintain because you understand what happens when you don't.

The Five Foundation Blocks of an Anti-Entropy Lifestyle

Reversing entropy isn't about finding one perfect solution. It is about consistently doing five things well and understanding that all five work together as a system rather than independently.

Picture these five things as five foundation blocks upon which a healthy anti-entropy lifestyle is built.

FIVE FOUNDATION BLOCKS OF AN ANTI-ENTROPY LIFESTYLE

1 REGULAR CHIROPRACTIC CARE

Remove nerve interference, restore proper spinal motion, and keep the nervous system running at full capacity. This is the foundation that allows your body to function at its best.

2 THERAPEUTIC MOVEMENT

Nourish discs, maintain mobility, activate stabilizers, and feed the brain the sensory input it needs to stay sharp and well-coordinated. Movement is a biological requirement that pushes back against entropy.

3 NERVOUS SYSTEM MANAGEMENT

Support the parasympathetic recovery state daily to reduce stress, balance your autonomic system, and promote healing and resilience. A managed nervous system heals better, recovers faster, and performs at a higher level.

4 SMART & HEALTHY NUTRITION

Fuel your body with anti-inflammatory foods and essential nutrients to support repair, reduce inflammation, and build strong, healthy tissues. You are what you give your body to build and repair with.

5 SLEEP

Deep, restorative sleep is when your body heals, repairs, and restores energy. Quality sleep is essential for recovery, hormonal balance, brain function, and long-term health.

These five foundation blocks work together to push back against entropy and build a stronger, more resilient you.

The first foundation block is regular chiropractic care. This is the foundation block that addresses the central cause of the breakdown this book has described from the beginning. Subluxations create nerve interference. Nerve interference degrades the function of every system the nervous system controls. Regular adjustments remove that interference, restore proper spinal motion, and keep the nervous system running at full capacity. Without this foundation block, the other four are working in a body whose master control system is operating below its potential.

The second foundation block is therapeutic movement. Not general exercise, though that matters too. Specific, intentional movement that keeps the spinal discs nourished through the imbibition cycle, maintains joint mobility, activates the deep stabilizers that protect the spine under load, and feeds the brain the rich sensory input it needs to stay sharp and well-coordinated. Movement is the biological requirement that no other intervention can replace, and doing it consistently is one of the most direct ways to push back against the entropy that's always working on your structural health.

The third foundation block is nervous system management. Your spine and your stress response are not separate systems. They are deeply connected, and the chronic sympathetic dominance that modern life creates compounds the physical interference that spinal dysfunction produces. Managing your nervous system means actively and deliberately supporting the parasympathetic recovery state through specific daily practices that shift the autonomic balance in the direction your body needs to heal, repair, and rebuild.

The fourth foundation block is smart and healthy nutrition. The body's ability to repair spinal structures, manage inflammation, and maintain the tissue quality that keeps the spine resilient depends on what you give it to work with. This doesn't require a dramatic dietary overhaul. It requires a few targeted choices that reduce the systemic inflammatory load and support the recovery and repair processes that happen in a healthy well-nourished body.

The fifth foundation block is sleep, good-quality restorative sleep. Deep restorative sleep is when your body heals and repairs after being in that sympathetic fight or flight phase. Parasympathetic activity promotes rest, digestion, and repair and recovery.

These five foundation blocks don't operate independently. They amplify each other. An adjustment works better in a body that moves daily. Movement produces better results in a nervous system that isn't locked in chronic sympathetic overdrive. Parasympathetic recovery is deeper and more restorative when the spine isn't generating mechanical stress signals that keep the sympathetic system partially activated. Nutrition supports all three by reducing the inflammatory environment that degrades spinal tissue and impairs nervous system function. Pull any one of these foundation blocks out and the other four become less effective. Keep all five in place consistently, and the compounding effect over months and years is genuinely remarkable.

The sections that follow build out each foundation block in specific, actionable detail. By the time you finish this chapter, you will have a complete daily blueprint that you can start implementing immediately, not someday, not next month, today.

Making Chiropractic Care a Non-Negotiable Part of Your Life

Most people approach chiropractic care the same way they approach a plumber. You call when something breaks. You stop calling when it's fixed. You don't think about it in between. That model produces exactly the outcomes you'd expect. The problem keeps coming back because the underlying conditions that created it were never fully addressed, and the maintenance that would prevent it from returning was never put in place.

The model that actually works is different. It is the dental hygiene model. You don't wait for a tooth to hurt before you brush. You don't skip cleanings until you're in agony. You maintain your teeth proactively because you understand that consistent maintenance prevents the breakdown that reactive treatment can never fully undo. The spine deserves exactly the same logic, and the stakes are higher, because the spine houses the nervous system that runs your entire body.

For most adults in reasonable spinal health who have completed a corrective care plan, monthly maintenance adjustments are the baseline. This frequency keeps the spine moving properly, catches new restrictions before they have time to compound into something significant, and maintains the nervous system function that every other aspect of your health depends on. If you're in a more physically demanding job, training hard, under significant stress, or in the middle of a corrective care phase, more frequent adjustments are appropriate. Your chiropractor can tell you about the right frequency for your specific situation. The key is that you have a schedule, you stick to it, and you don't use the absence of pain as a reason to cancel.

Cost is the most common barrier people cite, and it deserves a direct response. A monthly maintenance adjustment typically costs between sixty and one hundred dollars depending on your location and provider. That is lower than most medical doctor visit co-pays! Compare that to the cost of managing the chronic pain that develops when maintenance is skipped. A course of prescription pain medication. An MRI. A specialist consultation. An injection. Possibly surgery. The cost of doing nothing compounds in the same direction as the breakdown it fails to prevent. Monthly maintenance isn't an expense. It is the cheapest version of the care you'll eventually need anyway, paid proactively instead of reactively.

Time is the second barrier. A maintenance adjustment takes about fifteen to twenty minutes. Most people spend more time than that scrolling their phone before bed. The question isn't whether you have the time. The question is whether you've decided that your spine is worth the time. Scheduling your appointments in advance, three or four at a time, removes the weekly decision of whether to go. When it's already in the calendar, it gets treated like any other commitment that matters.

The "I feel fine" trap is the most dangerous barrier of all. As this book has established from the first chapter, feeling fine is not the same as being fine. Pain is a late signal. The degeneration and nerve interference that produce it have been building for months or years before they cross the threshold where you feel them. Waiting until you feel something to get adjusted is waiting until the cavity reaches the nerve before going to the dentist. By that point, the damage has already been done. Monthly maintenance catches the small restrictions before they become big problems. That is the whole point.

Here is a specific action to take today, not after you finish this chapter. Open your calendar right now and schedule your next three chiropractic appointments. If you don't have a chiropractor yet, block thirty minutes this week to research providers in your area, look for someone who offers a comprehensive initial assessment including postural analysis and spinal imaging, and book that assessment before the week is out. Three appointments scheduled in advance is the difference between a good intention and an actual plan.

The Daily Non-Negotiables — Small Habits That Compound Into Big Results

The gap between a body that ages gracefully and one that quietly falls apart isn't one dramatic choice. It is the accumulation of small daily decisions made consistently over time. The person who maintains their spinal health into their sixties and seventies didn't do anything heroic. They just did a handful of small things every day that most people either don't know about or don't bother with.

These are the daily non-negotiables. Each one is small enough to do without disrupting your life. Each one targets a specific mechanism in the anti-entropy system. And each one compounds over time in a way that no single dramatic intervention can replicate.

The first non-negotiable is the ten-minute morning mobility sequence we defined and discussed previously. Ten cat-cow movements, ten thoracic rotations per side, ten chin tucks, and two minutes of dead bugs. Done in that order, every morning, before you check your phone or do anything else. This sequence mobilizes the entire spine, stimulates the disc imbibition cycle, activates the deep stabilizers, and restores the cervical lordosis that forward head posture flattens overnight. It takes ten minutes. Set your alarm ten minutes earlier. Do it on the floor next to your bed so there's no friction between waking up and starting. The consistency of doing it first, before the day can crowd it out, is what makes it stick.

The second non-negotiable is the forty-five-minute movement break during your workday. Set a recurring timer on your phone. When it goes off, stand up for two minutes before sitting back down. Walk to get water, do ten slow shoulder rolls and neck stretches, or do ten hip hinges. Rotate through the three options so you're not doing the same movement repeatedly. This single habit prevents the sustained disc compression, deep stabilizer shutdown, and postural deterioration that accumulate during prolonged sitting. It takes sixteen minutes spread across an eight-hour workday. It costs nothing. And the cumulative effect on disc nutrition and spinal mechanics over months and years is significant.

The third non-negotiable is thirty minutes of walking every day. Not as a workout. As a spinal health practice. Walking loads the lumbar discs rhythmically through the imbibition cycle. It drives the thoracic rotation that keeps the mid-back mobile. It activates the gluteal muscles that are the primary dynamic stabilizers of the lumbar spine. It stimulates the proprioceptive input to the brain that keeps motor control precise. And it reduces cortisol and improves vagal tone in ways that directly support the parasympathetic recovery state. Morning, lunch, or evening, the timing matters less than the consistency. Schedule it the same way you schedule anything that matters.

The fourth non-negotiable is the five-minute diaphragmatic breathing practice every morning before you check your phone. Inhale for four counts through the nose, exhale for six to eight counts through the mouth. Five minutes. This activates the vagus nerve, shifts the nervous system from sympathetic toward parasympathetic, and sets the autonomic tone for the rest of the day in the direction your body needs. Research consistently shows that this practice produces measurable increases in heart rate variability that persist for hours after the practice ends. It costs nothing and requires no equipment. It just requires doing it before the day's demands override it.

The fifth non-negotiable is protecting your sleep environment. Keep your bedroom between 65 and 68 degrees Fahrenheit. No bright screens in the ninety minutes before bed. Sleep on your side with a pillow that keeps your cervical spine neutral and a pillow between your knees to keep your lumbar spine neutral. These three sleep habits directly reduce the mechanical and neurological inputs that prevent deep, restorative sleep. They don't require any additional time. They require specific, consistent choices in the environment where you already spend seven or eight hours every night.

The sixth non-negotiable is two targeted nutritional changes. Replace refined vegetable oils with olive oil or avocado oil. Add fatty fish twice a week or take a fish oil supplement providing at least two grams of combined EPA and DHA daily. These two changes reduce the systemic inflammatory load that accelerates spinal degeneration and impairs nervous system function. They don't require a dietary overhaul. They require two specific substitutions made consistently.

Six non-negotiables. None of them takes more than thirty minutes. Together, they address all five foundation blocks of the anti-entropy system every single day. The compounding effect of consistently following the six non-negotiables for three, four, five or six months produces changes in spinal health, energy, sleep quality, and nervous system function that are measurable, noticeable, and lasting. The compounding effect of skipping them consistently produces the opposite.

How to Stay Consistent When Life Gets in the Way

Knowing what to do is the easy part. Doing it when you're exhausted, traveling, stressed, or just not feeling motivated is where most plans fall apart. This section is about building the systems that make consistency the default rather than the exception.

The most important principle here is that motivation is unreliable and systems are not. You will not always feel like doing the morning mobility sequence. You will not always feel like taking the walk. There will be days when everything feels too hard and the path of least resistance is to skip it. If your plan depends on feeling motivated, it will fail on those days. If your plan is built into your environment and your schedule in a way that makes the right choice easier than the wrong one, it will survive those days.

Environment design is the most powerful tool for building consistency. Put your yoga mat next to your bed so the first thing you see when you wake up is the cue to do your morning sequence. Keep a foam roller visible in your living room rather than in a closet. Pack your walking shoes in your work bag the night before so there's no friction between deciding to walk at lunch and actually doing it. Fill your water bottle and leave it on your desk the night before so drinking enough water during the day doesn't require a decision. These aren't trivial details. Research on habit formation consistently shows that reducing the friction between intention and action is more effective at maintaining behavior than increasing motivation. Make the right choices easy and the wrong ones slightly harder, and your behavior changes without requiring willpower.

Traveling is one of the most common reasons people fall off their routines, and it deserves a specific plan rather than a vague intention to "try to keep up with things." Before any trip, identify the two non-negotiables you'll protect no matter what. The morning mobility sequence requires a floor and ten minutes. The diaphragmatic breathing requires nothing at all. These two habits can be done in any hotel room, any airport, any location in the world. Committing to protecting just these two during travel means that even your worst travel weeks don't completely break the chain. When you return, you're not starting over. You are picking up where you left off.

The two-day rule is one of the most practical consistency strategies available. Never miss two days in a row. One missed day is a pause. Two missed days is the beginning of a broken habit. When life genuinely prevents you from doing your full routine on a given day, do a reduced version rather than skipping entirely. Five minutes instead of ten. A ten-minute walk instead of thirty. One set of the morning sequence instead of the full routine. The reduced version keeps the chain intact and keeps the habit alive. It also makes it easier to return to the full version the next day because you haven't experienced the psychological reset of a complete break.

Progress tracking is the other major driver of consistency, and it's covered in detail in the next section. But the principle worth stating here is simple. What gets measured gets done. When you track your habits daily, even with nothing more than a checkmark in a notebook, you create a visual record of your consistency that becomes its own motivator. Seeing a streak of thirty consecutive days with checkmarks makes you significantly less likely to break that streak than you would be without the visual record. The tracking doesn't need to be sophisticated. It needs to be visible and done every day.

When you do fall off track, and at some point, you likely will, the most important thing is how quickly you recover. The people who maintain their anti-entropy plan over years aren't the ones who never slip. They are the ones who don't let a slip become a story. They don't spend days feeling guilty about missing a week of morning sequences. They do the sequence the next morning and move on. The gap between falling off and getting back on is the variable that determines long-term outcomes. Keep that gap as short as possible, and the occasional disruption becomes a minor blip rather than a permanent derailment.

One specific action that dramatically improves recovery speed after a disruption is scheduling your return in advance. Before a vacation, a busy work period, or any anticipated disruption to your routine, write down the specific date and the specific habit you'll restart when you return. "Monday morning, I restart the full morning sequence." That written commitment makes the return automatic rather than dependent on a decision made in the middle of the disruption when motivation is typically at its lowest.

Measuring Progress — How to Know It's Working

One of the most discouraging things about working on long-term health is that progress can be hard to see, especially when the goal is preventing something that hasn't happened yet. You can't see the disc degeneration that isn't progressing. You can't feel the nerve interference that isn't there. The absence of a bad outcome doesn't feel like a win, even when it absolutely is one.

This is why measuring the right things matters so much. Not just pain levels, though those matter. The full picture of how your body is functioning, across multiple dimensions, gives you the feedback loop you need to know whether your plan is working and where to adjust if it isn't.

Here are six specific metrics to track weekly. Each one can be rated on a simple one-to-ten scale. Each one reflects a different aspect of the anti-entropy system. Together, they give you a comprehensive picture of your progress that's far more useful than pain alone.

The first metric is morning stiffness. Rate how stiff you feel in the first fifteen minutes after waking up, where one is no stiffness at all and ten is severe stiffness that significantly limits your movement. This is one of the most sensitive indicators of spinal joint health and systemic inflammation. As your anti-entropy plan takes hold, this number should trend downward over weeks and months.

The second metric is afternoon energy. Rate your energy level at 3 PM on a typical day, where one is severely fatigued and ten is fully alert and energized. As previously covered, this metric is directly connected to nervous system function, and the background drain that spinal interference creates. Consistent improvement here reflects a nervous system that's spending less energy compensating and more energy performing.

The third metric is sleep quality. Rate how rested you feel when you wake up, where one is completely unrefreshed and ten is deeply restored. This reflects both the mechanical improvements in your sleep position and the autonomic shift toward parasympathetic recovery that consistent spinal care and nervous system management produce.

The fourth metric is range of motion. Once a week, perform three simple tests and note any changes. First, turn your head as far as you comfortably can to the right and then to the left, and note whether the range feels equal and full or restricted on either side. Second, try to touch your toes from a standing position with your knees straight and note how far you can reach. Third, clasp your hands behind your back from above and below and note whether one side is significantly more restricted than the other. These aren't precise clinical measurements. They're functional benchmarks that give you a consistent, repeatable picture of how your spinal mobility is changing over time.

The fifth metric is pain frequency and intensity. Not just whether you have pain today, but how often it shows up during the week and how intense it is when it does. Track this as two separate numbers: the number of days during the week when pain was present at a three or above, and the average intensity on those days. Over months of consistent anti-entropy practice, both numbers should trend downward. If they're not trending downward after six to eight weeks, that's information. Bring it to your chiropractor and have a specific conversation about what needs to be adjusted in your care plan.

The sixth metric is mental clarity and focus. Rate your cognitive sharpness during your most demanding work period of the day, where one is foggy and unfocused and ten is sharp and fully present. As the brain-body loop improves with better spinal health, this metric is often one of the first to show noticeable improvement, and it's one of the most motivating to track because the change in daily cognitive experience is immediately tangible.

Track these six metrics every Sunday evening. Write them in a notebook with the date. It takes five minutes. After four weeks, look at the trend across all six. After eight weeks, look again. After three months, compare your current averages to your starting point. The data you collect will be more compelling than anything written in this chapter, because it will be your own body's response measured in your own terms.

Beyond these weekly metrics, there are functional benchmarks worth tracking at the one-month, three-month, and six-month marks. At one month, you should notice that the morning mobility sequence feels easier and your range of motion in the three weekly tests has improved measurably. At three months, you should notice that the morning stiffness metric has dropped by at least two to three points from your starting baseline, and that your afternoon energy is consistently higher than it was when you started. At six months, you should notice that pain frequency has dropped significantly, that your sleep quality metric is consistently in the six-to-eight range, and that your chiropractor's assessment confirms measurable improvement in spinal alignment and range of motion compared to your initial findings.

If a metric isn't improving on this timeline, treat it as a signal rather than a failure. A morning stiffness score that isn't dropping after eight weeks of consistent care might mean the anti-inflammatory nutritional changes haven't been implemented fully. An afternoon energy score that isn't improving might mean the sleep environment changes haven't been made. A range of motion benchmark that isn't improving might mean the morning mobility sequence is being done inconsistently or that there's a specific spinal segment that needs more targeted attention in your care plan. The metrics don't just tell you how you're doing. They tell you where to look when things aren't moving in the right direction.

Progress in spinal health is rarely linear. There will be weeks where your numbers dip, often during periods of higher stress, disrupted sleep, or increased physical demand. A single bad week doesn't mean the plan isn't working. It means you're a human being living a real life. What matters is the trend over months, not the fluctuation over days. Keep tracking, keep showing up, and trust the compounding effect of consistent good choices made over time. That compounding is the most powerful force in your anti-entropy plan, and it works in your favor every single day that you put the inputs in.

Recap

Your anti-entropy plan is built on five foundation blocks: regular chiropractic care that keeps the nervous system running without interference, therapeutic movement that keeps the spine nourished and structurally resilient, nervous system management that protects the parasympathetic recovery state your body needs to heal, smart nutrition and recovery that reduce the inflammatory load and support healthy cell processes, and deep restorative sleep that fosters repair. All five blocks work together as a system. None of them works as well without the others.

The daily non-negotiables that power this plan are specific and small. The ten-minute morning mobility sequence. The forty-five-minute movement break. The thirty-minute walk. The five-minute breathing practice. The sleep environment corrections. The two targeted nutritional changes. None of them requires heroic effort. All of them compound over time into something that no single dramatic intervention can replicate.

Consistency is the variable that determines everything. Not perfection. Not intensity. Consistency. The systems and environment designs in this chapter exist specifically to make consistency easier than inconsistency, so that the right choices happen by default rather than by willpower. Build those systems, protect them during disruptions, and recover quickly when you fall off track.

Progress is real, measurable, and available to everyone who commits to the plan. Track the six weekly metrics. Watch the trends over months. Use the data your body gives you to refine your approach when something isn't moving in the right direction. The feedback loop you build through consistent tracking is what keeps the plan alive and effective over the long haul.

Four specific actions to take before you close this book.

First, write out your personal anti-entropy plan using the five foundation blocks as your framework. One page. Specific habits under each foundation block, specific frequencies, specific times of day. Make it concrete enough that you could hand it to someone else, and they'd know exactly what to do. Vague intentions don't survive contact with a busy week. A written, specific plan does.

Second, open your calendar right now and schedule your next three chiropractic appointments. If you don't have a chiropractor, block thirty minutes this week to find one and book an initial assessment. Do not wait until you're in pain. The whole point of this plan is that you don't need to be in pain to benefit from it.

Third, choose two of the six daily non-negotiables from this chapter and commit to them for the next thirty days without missing a day. Just two. The morning mobility sequence and the daily walk are the highest-return starting point for most people. Do those two every day for thirty days, track them with a simple checkmark in a notebook, and let the results show you what's possible before you add more.

Fourth, set up your weekly Sunday check-in. Five minutes, six metrics, written in a notebook. Do it at the same time every week so it becomes automatic. After four weeks, review the trends. After three months, compare your current numbers to where you started. That comparison will tell you more about what this plan is doing for your body than anything else in this chapter.

Entropy is always working. That hasn't changed and it won't change. But so is your ability to push back against it, and every good choice you make from this point forward is a deposit into the account that keeps your body functioning, moving, and feeling the way it was designed to. That account builds slowly, quietly, and cumulatively, the same way entropy tears things down. The difference is that you're the one deciding which direction it goes.

Conclusion

The Big Picture — What You Now Know That Most People Never Will

You started this book with a feeling. Maybe it was the stiffness that greets you every morning before your body finally loosens up. Maybe it was the fatigue that doesn't fully lift no matter how much you sleep. Maybe it was a quiet, nagging sense that something was slowly going wrong, that the aches and the low energy and the reduced range of motion weren't just normal aging but something worth paying attention to. That feeling was right. And now you understand why.

"Get the Big Idea and all else follows."

—B.J. Palmer

Entropy is real. It has been working on your body since long before you ever felt a thing. Your spine has been responding to every hour of sitting, every posture held too long, every movement skipped, every subluxation that went uncorrected. The breakdown doesn't announce itself. It compounds quietly, in increments too small to notice on any given day, until one morning the stiffness takes longer to clear or the pain crosses a threshold you can no longer explain away. By that point, the process has been running for years.

That is the part most people never learn.

They live their whole lives using pain as their measuring stick for health. No pain means everything is fine. Pain means something broke. So, they wait. They manage. They take something for it and hope it passes. And the whole time, entropy keeps working in the background, winning ground that gets harder and harder to recover the longer it goes unaddressed. The gap between how a person feels and how their spine is actually doing can be enormous, and most people spend decades in that gap without ever knowing it exists.

You know it exists now. And that changes everything.

You understand that your nervous system is the master controller of every function in your body. Your heart rate, your immune response, your digestion, your sleep, your mood, your cognitive sharpness, all of it runs on signals that travel through the spinal cord and out through the nerve roots that branch off at every level of your spine. When the spine is healthy, aligned, and moving properly, those signals travel without interference, and the body runs the way it was designed to. When the spine breaks down, the signals get compressed, distorted, and weakened, and the effects ripple out into every system the nervous system controls. That is not a back problem. That is a whole-body problem with a spinal cause.

You understand innate intelligence now, the body's built-in capacity to heal, regulate, and restore itself when the nervous system is free from interference. Your body hasn't turned against you. It has been trying to do its job the entire time. The pain, the fatigue, the dysfunction you've been experiencing isn't your body failing. It is your body working as hard as it can under conditions that are making its job harder than it should be. Remove the interference, restore the conditions the body needs, and the intelligence that's been there your whole life can finally do what it was designed to do at full capacity.

You understand the history of chiropractic care, where it came from, why it was fought, and how thoroughly it's been validated by over a century of clinical practice and research. You know that spinal manipulation isn't a fringe idea or a party trick. It is a well-documented, rigorously studied intervention that restores joint motion, floods the nervous system with sensory input it had been missing, shifts the autonomic balance toward parasympathetic recovery, and produces measurable changes in brain function within seconds of the adjustment. You know that every NFL team has a chiropractor on staff not because of ideology but because the results are too consistent to ignore.

You understand the difference between sympathetic overdrive and parasympathetic recovery, and why the balance between those two states determines whether your body is breaking down or building back up. You understand that poor spinal health doesn't just cause back pain. It keeps the sympathetic system partially activated around the clock through mechanical stress signals the brain interprets as a constant low-grade threat, and that this sustained activation suppresses the very healing systems your body needs to repair what daily life breaks down. Sleep suffers. Immunity suffers. Digestion suffers. Energy suffers. And the person experiencing all of that rarely connects it to their spine because none of it feels like a back problem.

You understand spinal degeneration, what it actually looks like at the structural level, how it progresses through stages, how it starts silently in early adulthood and compounds for decades before most people receive a diagnosis. You know that earlier is always better, that stages one and two are where the game is won or lost, and that the people who halt the progression and partially reverse the damage are the ones who stopped waiting for pain to tell them something was wrong.

You understand the three milestones of recovery. Return to work. Return to play. Return to full function. You know that stopping at the first milestone because the pain went away is like stopping a course of antibiotics because you feel better. The symptom responded. The underlying problem didn't. The people who reach full function are the ones who understood this before the pain went away and stayed the course because of it.

You understand the inside-out model of health, and why removing the cause produces fundamentally different results than managing the symptom. You know when outside-in treatment makes sense and when it's being used to manage a problem that has a solvable root cause. You know the question to ask about every health decision: is this addressing why my body is struggling, or is it managing what my body is experiencing because of why it's struggling?

And you have the anti-entropy plan. The five foundation blocks. The six daily non-negotiables. The six weekly metrics. The systems that make consistency easier than inconsistency. The framework for measuring your progress in terms that actually reflect how your body is functioning rather than just whether something hurts today.

Most people will never have this picture. They will manage symptoms their whole lives without ever understanding the system those symptoms are coming from. They will accept the stiffness, the fatigue, the reduced function as the inevitable cost of getting older, never knowing that entropy can be slowed, stopped, and in many cases reversed when the right care is applied consistently and early enough. They will reach their sixties and seventies wondering why their body feels like it's working against them, not realizing that the body they have is largely the result of the daily inputs they gave it over decades.

You have a different picture now. That is not a small thing. That is the difference between being a passenger in your own health and being the driver.

The Moment That Changes Everything — Take Action Today

Reading this book was a real first step. Understanding entropy, the nervous system, spinal degeneration, innate intelligence, the inside-out model, the recovery roadmap, all of it matters. Knowledge is the foundation. But it's only the foundation. A foundation without a structure built on top of it is just a slab of concrete sitting in a field. It doesn't become anything until someone starts building.

The readers who get their lives back are not the ones who understood the most. They are the ones who did something with what they understood. They are the ones who booked the appointment instead of thinking about booking it. They are the ones who started the morning sequence instead of planning to start it next week when things slow down. They are the ones who showed up to their follow-up appointments even after the pain went away, because they understood that the pain going away wasn't the finish line.

Here is what "next week when things slow down" actually means in practice. It means never. Life doesn't slow down. The demands don't reduce themselves. The calendar doesn't magically clear. The window you're waiting for doesn't open on its own. The people who wait for the perfect conditions to start taking care of their spine are the same people who, five years from now, are dealing with stage two or stage three degeneration that would have been stage one if they'd started when they first had the information to act on.

The version of you that wakes up without stiffness, that moves through the day with real energy, that sleeps deeply and wakes up restored, that thinks clearly in the afternoon instead of pushing through fog, that does the physical things you love without bracing for the consequences, that version isn't a fantasy. It is a description of what happens when the spine is maintained, the nervous system is running without interference, and the daily habits that support both are in place consistently. That version is achievable. The research supports it. The clinical outcomes confirm it. The only variable is whether you act on what you now know.

Not next week. Today.

Today means one specific thing done before you go to sleep tonight. Not a list of ten things. One. The single most important action you can take right now is to schedule a comprehensive spinal assessment with a qualified chiropractor. Not a quick look and an adjustment. A full assessment that includes postural analysis, range of motion testing, orthopedic and neurological evaluation, and spinal imaging if indicated. This gives you the actual information about your spine that everything else in your plan depends on. You can't make good decisions about your spinal health without knowing your starting point. The assessment gives you that starting point. Everything else builds from there.

If you already have a chiropractor, your one action today is to call and schedule your next appointment, or the next three if you've been inconsistent. Put them in your calendar before you close this book. Treat them the way you'd treat a meeting you can't move, because in terms of what they do for your long-term health, they matter more than most meetings you'll ever attend.

If the assessment reveals that your spine is in better shape than you had expected, that's genuinely good news and it means your maintenance plan is about keeping it that way. If it reveals degeneration, or subluxations you didn't know were there, that's also good news, because you caught it with information rather than waiting for it to catch you with pain. Either way, the assessment gives you what you need to move forward with clarity instead of guesswork.

The people who change their health don't do it because they finally found enough motivation. Motivation comes and goes. They do it because they made a specific decision, at a specific moment, to act on what they knew instead of filing it away for later. This is that moment. What you do with it is up to you.

Your Step-by-Step Roadmap — Everything You Need to Start Right Now

Everything in this book, every concept, every explanation, every chapter, points toward this. A clear, specific, actionable sequence you can follow starting today. Not a collection of vague suggestions. A roadmap with real steps, in the right order, with real outcomes attached to each one.

Step one: accept that entropy is real and that your body is always moving in one direction. There is no neutral gear. Every day you're either pushing back against the breakdown or letting it win a little more ground. That's not meant to create anxiety. It's meant to create clarity. You are not a passive victim of aging. You are an active participant in the direction your body is moving, and you have far more influence over that direction than most people ever realize. Start from that position.

Step two: stop waiting for pain before you act. Pain is a late signal. By the time it shows up reliably, the underlying problem has usually been building for months, sometimes years. The cost of waiting for pain is the compounding damage that accumulates while you're waiting. Get a spinal assessment now, not when something hurts badly enough to force you into it. The earlier the assessment, the more options you have. The more options you have, the better the outcomes available to you.

Step three: find a qualified chiropractor and commit to a care plan, not just a single visit. One adjustment is like one workout. It does something, but it doesn't change anything by itself. The spine responds to repetition. The nervous system learns from consistent input. A care plan that moves you through the relief phase, the corrective phase, and into maintenance is what produces the lasting results that a single visit can only hint at. Ask your chiropractor which phase you're in, what the goals of that phase are, and what the criteria are for moving to the next one. Know where you are on the map at all times.

Step four: learn your nervous system and protect it like the master controller it is. Your nervous system runs everything. Every function in your body depends on the quality of the signals traveling through the spinal cord and out through the nerve roots at every level of your spine. When those signals are clear, the body functions at its best. When they're compressed or distorted, the effects show up everywhere, often in places you'd never connect to your spine. Your spine isn't just about your back. It is about the quality of the communication network that runs your entire body. Treat it accordingly.

Step five: balance your sympathetic and parasympathetic systems every single day. The five-minute diaphragmatic breathing practice every morning. The daily walk that reduces cortisol and improves vagal tone. The sleep environment corrections that protect the deep, restorative sleep stages where real repair happens. The consistent chiropractic care that removes the mechanical stress signals keeping your sympathetic system partially activated around the clock. These aren't separate habits for separate reasons. They are all inputs into the same system, and they compound together into a nervous system that spends more time in the healing state and less time in the survival state.

Step six: move your body every day in ways that feed your spine. The ten-minute morning mobility sequence. The forty-five-minute movement break during your workday. The thirty-minute daily walk. The progressive resistance training that rebuilds the structural strength the spine needs to hold its alignment under the demands of real life. Your discs don't have a blood supply. They eat through movement. Stop moving and they stop eating. Start moving consistently and they start recovering. It is that direct.

Step seven: set your sights on full function, not just pain relief, and track your progress along the way. Pain relief is the floor, not the ceiling. Full function means doing everything you want to do, at the level you want to do it, without your spine or nervous system being the limiting factor. Write down specifically what full function looks like for you. The activities you want to return to. The energy level you want to have. The physical demands you want to meet without limitation. Make it concrete. Track the six weekly metrics previously covered. Watch the trends over months. Use the data to refine your plan and to remind yourself, on the hard days, that the direction is right even when the progress feels slow.

Step eight: build your five-foundation block anti-entropy lifestyle and make it non-negotiable. 1. Regular chiropractic care. 2. Therapeutic movement. 3. Nervous system management. 4. Smart nutrition. 5. Restorative sleep. All five, consistently, working as a system. Not perfectly. Consistently. The compounding effect of consistent good inputs over months and years is the most powerful force available to you in the fight against entropy, and it works in your favor every single day that you put the inputs in.

That is the roadmap. Eight steps. Each one builds on the one before it. Each one moves you further from breakdown and closer to the full, functional, energized version of your health that this book has been pointing toward from the first page.

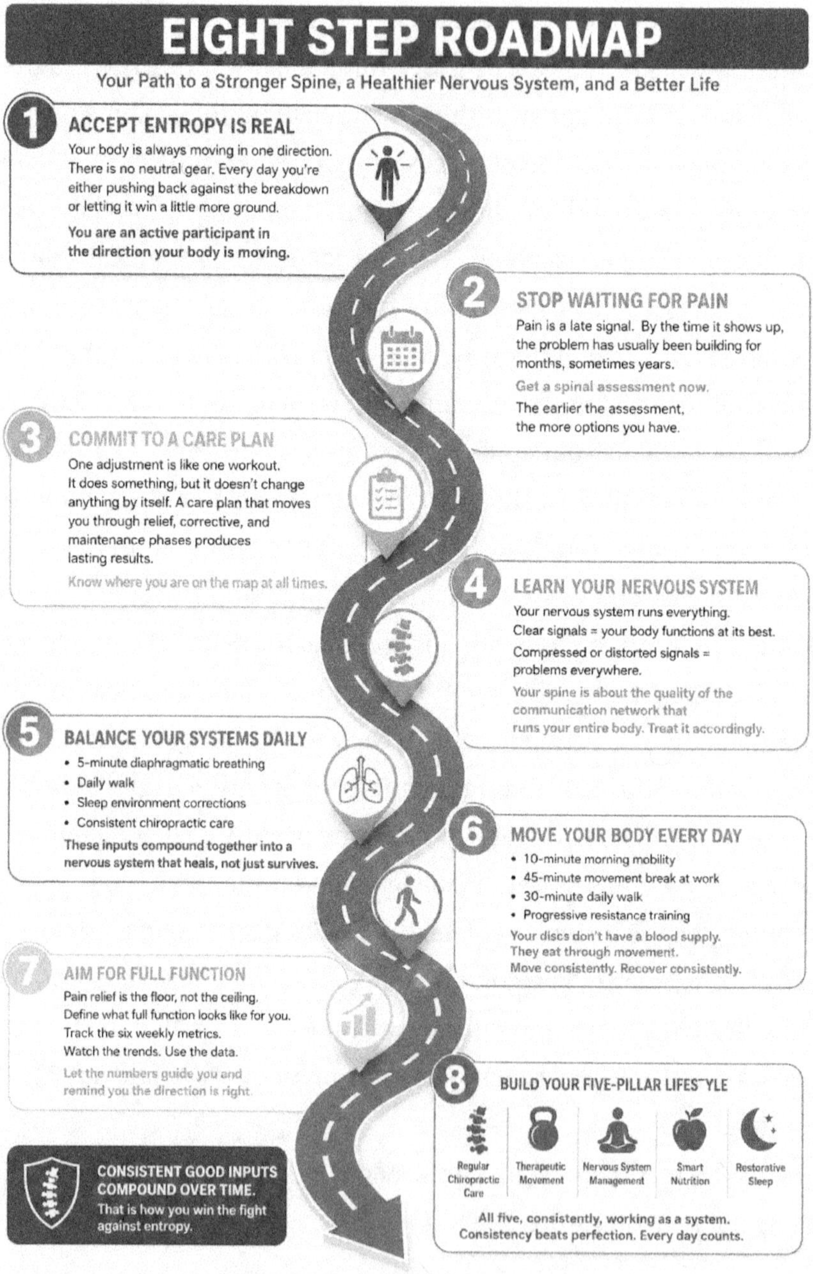

Life is genuinely better adjusted! Not just with less pain, though there will be less pain. With more energy. Better sleep. Sharper thinking. A body that shows up fully for the moments that actually matter. A nervous system running at the capacity it was designed for. A spine that's being maintained instead of slowly abandoned. That is the real promise of everything in these pages, and it's available to you at any age, from any starting point, as long as you're willing to start.

The entropy is real. So is your ability to push back against it. Start today.

"He who has health has hope, and he who has hope has everything."

—Arabian Proverb

Glossary of Terms

✦✦✦

Activator (Activator method)
A small, handheld chiropractic instrument that delivers a quick, controlled, low-force impulse to a specific spinal segment or joint. The tool and the method are used as an alternative to manual adjusting techniques to help improve spinal segment or joint motion.

Adjustment (Chiropractic adjustment)
A precise, controlled force delivered to a specific spinal joint to restore normal joint motion, reduce nerve interference, and improve nervous system function. Throughout this book, the chiropractic adjustment is presented as the central therapeutic intervention for improving spinal health and supporting the body's natural healing abilities.

Adrenal Cortex
The outer portion of the adrenal gland that produces cortisol and other hormones involved in the body's response to stress. This book discusses its role in the physiological stress response initiated by the hypothalamus.

Adrenal Medulla
The inner portion of the adrenal gland that releases epinephrine and

norepinephrine during activation of the sympathetic nervous system, preparing the body for the fight-or-flight response.

Afferent Input

Sensory information traveling from the body to the brain. This book explains that healthy spinal motion continually supplies the brain with afferent information that helps maintain coordination, posture, and normal nervous system function.

Alignment

The proper structural relationship of the vertebrae and other joints that allows efficient movement and optimal nervous system communication.

Amygdala

A structure within the brain involved in processing emotions and perceived threats. This book describes it as part of the pathway that initiates the body's stress response.

Anti-Entropy Lifestyle

The collection of daily habits described in this book—including chiropractic care, therapeutic movement, stress management, nutrition, and sleep and recovery—that work together to counter the body's natural tendency toward degeneration.

Anti-inflammatory Diet

A nutritional approach emphasizing foods that help regulate inflammation while minimizing foods that promote chronic inflammatory processes.

Antacid

A medication used to neutralize stomach acid. This book uses antacids as an example of treating symptoms without necessarily addressing underlying causes.

Atlas (C1)

The first cervical vertebra (C1), located directly beneath the skull. It supports the head and plays an important role in upper cervical motion.

Autonomic Nervous System

The division of the nervous system responsible for automatic body functions such as heart rate, digestion, blood pressure, and respiration. It includes the sympathetic and parasympathetic nervous systems.

B.J. Palmer

Bartlett Joshua Palmer, son of D.D. Palmer, who expanded chiropractic education, promoted research, and helped establish chiropractic as a recognized healthcare profession.

Brain-Body Loop

The continuous two-way communication between the brain and the body through the nervous system. This book emphasizes that healthy spinal function supports this ongoing exchange of information.

Brain Fog

A non-medical term used to describe reduced mental clarity, poor concentration, or slowed thinking. This book discusses it as a possible manifestation of altered nervous system function.

Cavitation

The audible popping sound that may occur during a chiropractic adjustment, produced by rapid gas release within synovial fluid. The sound itself is a by-product rather than the objective of the adjustment.

Cerebellum

The portion of the brain responsible for balance, posture, coordination, muscle tone, and refinement of movement. This book explains its close relationship with sensory input from the spine.

Central Nervous System

The brain and spinal cord, which together serve as the body's primary control and communication center.

Cervical Lordosis

The normal forward curvature of the cervical spine. This book discusses restoration of cervical lordosis as part of correcting forward head posture.

Chiropractic

A healthcare profession centered on restoring spinal function and optimizing nervous system performance through chiropractic adjustments and related conservative care.

Chronic Stress

Persistent activation of the body's stress response that can impair healing, increase inflammation, and contribute to long-term dysfunction.

Cortisol

A hormone released by the adrenal cortex during stress. It helps the body respond to immediate demands but may contribute to health problems when chronically elevated.

D.D. Palmer

Daniel David Palmer, founder of chiropractic, who performed the first chiropractic adjustment in 1895 and introduced the concepts of vertebral subluxation and innate intelligence as presented in this book.

Degenerative Disc Disease

The gradual deterioration of one or more intervertebral discs characterized by loss of hydration, reduced disc height, and diminished shock-absorbing capacity. The book describes it as a progressive consequence of entropy that may be slowed through appropriate care and maintenance.

Degenerative Joint Disease

Progressive deterioration of the joints associated with cartilage wear, reduced mobility, and structural changes over time.

Digestion

The process of breaking down food into absorbable nutrients. This book explains that digestive function is influenced by the autonomic nervous system.

Disc Imbibition

The natural process by which intervertebral discs absorb water and nutrients during alternating cycles of loading and unloading created by movement.

Docosahexaenoic Acid (DHA)

An omega-3 fatty acid discussed as part of nutritional strategies that support nervous system health and help regulate inflammation.

Edwin Smith Papyrus

An ancient Egyptian medical text describing trauma, spinal injuries, neurological observations, and manual treatment techniques that are discussed as historical foundations related to chiropractic principles.

Energy

Within the discussion of entropy, the input required to maintain or improve biological systems. This book uses movement, nutrition, chiropractic care, and healthy habits as examples of energy applied against breakdown.

Entropy

The Second Law of Thermodynamics describing the natural tendency of systems to move toward disorder. The central theme of this book uses entropy to explain aging, degeneration, and the need for continual maintenance of the body.

Eicosapentaenoic Acid (EPA)

An omega-3 fatty acid presented as part of an anti-inflammatory nutritional approach supporting overall health.

Epinephrine

A hormone and neurotransmitter released from the adrenal medulla during activation of the sympathetic nervous system, helping prepare the body for immediate action.

Fastigial Nucleus

A deep cerebellar nucleus involved in balance, posture, muscle tone, and autonomic regulation. This book describes it as part of neurological pathways influenced by spinal adjustments.

Fight-or-Flight Response

The body's automatic survival response mediated primarily by the sympathetic nervous system, increasing alertness, heart rate, blood pressure, and stress hormone release.

Foraminal Stenosis

Narrowing of the openings through which spinal nerves exit the vertebral column, potentially contributing to nerve irritation.

Forward Head Posture

A postural distortion in which the head shifts anterior to its normal position, substantially increasing mechanical stress on the cervical spine.

Function

The ability of the body or one of its systems to operate efficiently. Throughout this book, restoration of normal function is emphasized over simply reducing symptoms.

Georg Ebers Papyrus

An ancient Egyptian medical papyrus discussed in the manuscript for its descriptions of anatomy, musculoskeletal conditions, manual therapies, and concepts that parallel later chiropractic principles.

Glucosamine

A naturally occurring amino sugar commonly used as a nutritional supplement to support cartilage and joint health. This book cites glucosamine as one example of providing the body with the resources needed to counteract entropy and support degenerative joints.

Gray Matter

The portions of the brain and spinal cord containing nerve cell bodies where information is processed and integrated.

Headache

Pain or discomfort involving the head or upper neck. This book notes that some headaches may originate from dysfunction of the cervical spine and nervous system.

Healing

The body's natural process of repairing damaged tissues and restoring function. Throughout this book, healing is presented as an innate biological process that depends on healthy nervous system communication.

Hippocrates

The Greek physician widely regarded as the Father of Medicine. This book discusses his historical emphasis on the importance of the spine in health and disease.

Homeostasis

The body's ability to maintain a stable internal environment despite continual changes within and outside the body.

Hypertonicity

Excessive muscle tension or increased resting muscle tone that may accompany joint dysfunction or injury.

Hypothalamus

A small region of the brain that regulates numerous automatic body functions and serves as the primary control center for initiating the physiological stress response.

Ibuprofen

A nonsteroidal anti-inflammatory medication referenced in this book as an example of temporarily treating symptoms without necessarily correcting their underlying cause.

Immune System

The body's defense system against infection and disease. This book explains that nervous system function influences immune regulation and overall health.

Inflammation

The body's protective response to injury or irritation. Acute inflammation supports healing, whereas chronic inflammation contributes to tissue breakdown and degenerative change.

Innate Intelligence

A foundational chiropractic concept describing the body's inherent ability to regulate, organize, repair, and heal itself through the nervous system when communication pathways remain unobstructed.

Interference

A disruption of normal communication within the nervous system. In chiropractic terminology, interference may reduce the body's ability to regulate function and maintain health.

Intermediolateral Nucleus

A column of nerve cell bodies within the lateral gray matter of the spinal cord from T1 through L2 that contains sympathetic preganglionic neurons involved in autonomic regulation.

Intervertebral Disc

The fibrocartilaginous structure located between adjacent vertebrae that functions as a shock absorber while permitting movement and distributing mechanical loads through the spine.

Joint Fixation

A restriction or loss of normal joint motion. This book describes fixation as a target for chiropractic adjustment because restricted spinal joints may alter movement and nervous system function.

Joint Dysfunction

Abnormal movement or mechanical function of a joint that may contribute to pain, stiffness, reduced mobility, or altered neurological input.

Ligament

A strong band of connective tissue that connects bone to bone and helps stabilize joints, including the joints of the spine.

Ligaplex

A nutritional supplement available from Standard Process referenced in this book as part of supporting connective tissue and joint health within an anti-entropy approach to maintaining the body.

Lordosis

The normal forward curvature of the cervical and lumbar spine. Maintaining healthy spinal curves is presented as an important component of proper posture and spinal biomechanics.

Lumbar Spine

The lower portion of the vertebral column consisting of five lumbar vertebrae. The lumbar spine bears much of the body's weight and is commonly affected by degeneration, injury, and mechanical stress.

Lungs

The primary organs of respiration. This book notes that nervous system communication influences the function of every organ system, including the lungs.

Macrophage

A type of white blood cell involved in removing damaged tissue, debris, and microorganisms. This book references macrophages as part of the body's natural healing process.

Mechanoreceptor

A specialized sensory receptor located in joints, muscles, tendons, and ligaments that detects movement, pressure, and position. This book emphasizes the abundance of mechanoreceptors within the spine and their importance in providing sensory input to the brain.

Medulla Oblongata

The lower portion of the brainstem that helps regulate essential automatic functions such as breathing, heart rate, and blood pressure.

Mobility

The ability of a joint or body region to move through its normal range of motion. Maintaining spinal mobility is presented as essential for healthy nervous system function.

Movement

A fundamental biological requirement for maintaining healthy joints, muscles, discs, and nervous system function. Throughout this book, purposeful movement is described as one of the body's primary defenses against entropy.

Multifidus

A deep spinal stabilizing muscle that supports vertebral alignment and contributes to spinal stability during movement.

Muscle Spindle

A sensory receptor located within skeletal muscle that detects changes in muscle length and contributes to posture, balance, coordination, and reflex activity.

Neuroplasticity

The nervous system's ability to adapt, reorganize, and modify its structure and function throughout life in response to experience, movement, and sensory input.

Norepinephrine

A neurotransmitter and hormone released during sympathetic nervous system activation that increases alertness, heart rate, and blood pressure as part of the body's stress response.

Nucleus Pulposus

The gel-like central portion of an intervertebral disc that distributes compressive forces and contributes to the disc's shock-absorbing function.

Nutrition

The intake of nutrients required for growth, tissue repair, energy production, and maintenance of normal body function. This book identifies proper nutrition as one of the foundations of an anti-entropy lifestyle.

Omega-3 Fatty Acids

Essential polyunsaturated fats, including EPA and DHA, discussed in this book for their role in supporting normal inflammatory regulation and overall health.

Orthopedics

The branch of healthcare concerned with the diagnosis and treatment of disorders affecting bones, joints, muscles, ligaments, tendons, and related structures.

Osteoarthritis

A degenerative joint disorder characterized by progressive cartilage deterioration, joint stiffness, and reduced mobility. This book discusses osteoarthritis as one manifestation of long-term structural degeneration.

Parasympathetic Nervous System

The division of the autonomic nervous system responsible for rest, digestion, recovery, and healing. This book describes activation of this system as essential for repair and long-term health.

Physical Therapy

A healthcare profession focused on restoring movement, strength, mobility, and function through therapeutic exercise and rehabilitation. This book describes physical therapy as complementary to chiropractic care during recovery.

Pontomedullary Reticular Formation

A region of the brainstem involved in regulating posture, muscle tone, autonomic activity, and arousal. This book discusses it as part of neurological pathways influenced by spinal adjustments.

Posture

The alignment and positioning of the body during standing, sitting, and movement. Healthy posture reduces unnecessary stress on the spine and supports efficient nervous system function.

Prefrontal Cortex

The front portion of the brain responsible for executive function, judgment, planning, attention, and emotional regulation. This book discusses research demonstrating changes in prefrontal cortex activity following spinal adjustments.

Proprioception

The body's awareness of the position and movement of its joints and limbs. Continuous proprioceptive input from the spine helps the brain coordinate posture, balance, and movement.

Quadratus Lumborum

A deep muscle of the lower back that stabilizes the lumbar spine and assists with side bending and trunk control. Hypertonicity of this muscle is discussed in clinical examples within this book.

Range of Motion

The amount of movement available at a joint or body region. Restoring normal range of motion is presented as one of the primary goals of chiropractic adjustments and rehabilitation.

Rehabilitation

A structured program of therapeutic exercise and functional training designed to restore strength, mobility, coordination, and normal movement following injury or dysfunction. This book emphasizes rehabilitation alongside chiropractic care for lasting results.

Reticular Formation

A network of interconnected neurons within the brainstem that helps regulate consciousness, muscle tone, posture, autonomic activity, and sensory processing.

Return to Function

The restoration of normal physical capability and performance in daily life. This book identifies return to function as the ultimate goal of successful care rather than simply reducing pain.

Return to Play

The safe resumption of recreational or athletic activities following injury or treatment after adequate healing and functional recovery.

Return to Work

The ability to safely resume occupational duties following injury or illness with sufficient strength, mobility, and function.

Recovery

The biological and functional process through which the body repairs tissue, restores normal movement, and returns toward optimal health following injury, illness, or dysfunction.

Second Law of Thermodynamics

A fundamental law of physics stating that systems naturally move toward greater disorder over time unless energy is applied. This book uses this law to explain entropy and the body's tendency toward degeneration without proper maintenance.

Sensory Afference

The continuous flow of sensory information traveling from the body to the brain. This book emphasizes that healthy spinal movement provides essential afferent input for optimal brain function.

Serotonin

A chemical messenger (neurotransmitter) that helps regulate mood, sleep, appetite, digestion, memory, and overall well-being. It also plays an important role in communication between nerve cells throughout the brain and body.

Spinal Adjustment

A specific chiropractic procedure in which a controlled force is applied to a spinal joint to restore normal motion, reduce nerve interference, and improve nervous system function.

Spinal Cord

The major communication pathway between the brain and the rest of the body, protected by the vertebral column and responsible for transmitting sensory and motor information.

Spinal Degeneration

The progressive structural deterioration of the spine involving discs, joints, ligaments, and supporting tissues over time.

Spinal Manipulation

A manual therapeutic procedure that restores movement to restricted spinal joints. This book identifies the chiropractic adjustment as a specific form of spinal manipulation.

Spinal Nerve

One of the paired nerves that exits the spinal cord through openings between adjacent vertebrae to supply sensation and motor function throughout the body.

Spine

Also called the vertebral column, the central structural support of the body that protects the spinal cord while allowing flexibility, stability, and movement.

Stress

The body's physical and emotional response to real or perceived challenges. This book explains how chronic stress influences the nervous system, hormones, inflammation, and overall health.

Subluxation

A chiropractic term describing a vertebral dysfunction or misalignment that may interfere with normal joint motion and nervous system communication.

Sympathetic Nervous System

The division of the autonomic nervous system responsible for the fight-or-flight response and increased physiological readiness during stress.

Synovial Fluid

The lubricating fluid found within synovial joints that nourishes cartilage, reduces friction, and facilitates smooth joint movement.

Synovium

The specialized membrane lining synovial joints that produces synovial fluid to lubricate and nourish the joint.

Therapeutic Movement

Purposeful movement prescribed to improve joint mobility, disc nutrition, muscular stability, posture, and nervous system function.

Thoracic Spine

The middle portion of the vertebral column consisting of twelve vertebrae that articulate with the ribs and contribute to trunk stability and mobility.

Transversus Abdominis

A deep abdominal muscle that functions as a primary stabilizer of the lumbar spine and core during movement.

Tribonucleation

The technical term describing the rapid formation and collapse of gas bubbles within synovial fluid that produces the audible popping sound sometimes heard during joint cavitation.

Vertebra

One of the individual bones that make up the spinal column. Together, the vertebrae protect the spinal cord while providing support, flexibility, and movement.

Vertebral Column

Also known as the spine, the vertebral column is the central structural support of the body composed of 33 vertebrae, intervertebral discs, ligaments, and joints that protect the spinal cord and allow movement.

Vertebral Dysfunction

Abnormal motion or mechanical function of a vertebral segment. This book describes vertebral dysfunction as a potential source of altered biomechanics and nervous system interference.

White Blood Cell

A cell of the immune system responsible for helping defend the body against infection and participating in tissue repair. This book discusses immune cells as part of the body's innate healing processes.

Wilk v. AMA

The landmark antitrust lawsuit in which chiropractors successfully challenged the American Medical Association's organized efforts to restrict the chiropractic profession. The case is presented as a pivotal event in the acceptance of chiropractic within mainstream healthcare.

X-ray

A diagnostic imaging technique that uses electromagnetic radiation to visualize bones and other structures. This book discusses X-rays as part of a comprehensive chiropractic evaluation when clinically indicated.

References

✦✦✦

1. Clausius R. (1865). Ueber verschiedene für die Anwendung bequeme Formen der Hauptgleichungen der mechanischen Wärmetheorie [Concerning several conveniently applicable forms for the main equations of the mechanical heat theory]. Annalen der Physik, 201(7), 353–400. ↑
2. Cramer SC, Sur SR, Dobkin BH, et al. (2011). Harnessing neuroplasticity for clinical applications. Brain, 134(6), 1591–1609. ↑
3. Coronado RA, Gay CW, Bialosky JE, Carnaby GD, Bishop MD, George SZ. (2012). Changes in pain sensitivity following spinal manipulation: A systematic review and meta-analysis. Journal of Electromyography and Kinesiology, 22(5), 752–767. ↑
4. Millan, M, Leboeuf-Yde C, Budgell B & Amorim M. (2012). The effect of spinal manipulative therapy on spinal range of motion: A systematic literature review. Chiropractic and Manual Therapy. 2012 Aug 6;20(1):23.↑
5. Ebbell B (1937). The Papyrus Ebers: The greatest Egyptian medical document. Copenhagen: Levin & Munksgaard. ↑

6. Breasted JH, New-York Historical Society (1930). The Edwin Smith surgical papyrus. Chicago, Ill: The University of Chicago Press. ↑
7. Johnson CD & Green BN (2021). Looking back at the lawsuit that transformed the chiropractic profession, part 7: Lawsuit and decisions. Journal of Chiropractic Education, 35(Suppl. 1), 97–116. ↑
8. Shekelle PG, Alan HA, Chassin MR, Hurwitz E, Park RE, Phillips RB, and Brook R. (1992) The Appropriateness of Spinal Manipulation for Low-Back Pain: Indications and Ratings by an All-Chiropractic Expert Panel. Santa Monica, CA: RAND Corporation. ↑
9. Meade TW, Dyer SB, Townsend W, and Frank AO. (1990). Low back pain of mechanical origin: Randomised comparison of chiropractic and hospital outpatient treatment. BMJ, 300(6737), 1431–1437. ↑
10. Meade TW, Dyer SB and Frank, AO (1995). Randomised comparison of chiropractic and hospital outpatient management for low back pain: Results from extended follow up. BMJ, 311(7001), 349–351. ↑
11. Thornton JS, Caneiro JP, Hartvigsen J, Ardern CL, et al (2021). Treating low back pain in athletes: A systematic review with meta-analysis. British Journal of Sports Medicine, 55(12), 656–662. ↑
12. Lisi AJ, Goertz C, Lawrence DJ and Satyanarayana P. (2009). Characteristics of Veterans Health Administration chiropractors and chiropractic clinics. Journal of Rehabilitation Research & Development, 46(8), 997–1002. ↑
13. Haavik H, Niazi IK, Jochumsen M, Sherwin D, Flavel S and Türker KS. (2017). Impact of spinal manipulation on cortical drive to upper and lower limb muscles. Brain Sciences, 7(1), Article 2. ↑
14. Taylor HH and Murphy B. (2008). Altered sensorimotor integration with cervical spine manipulation. Journal of Manipulative and Physiological Therapeutics, 31(2), 115–126. ↑
15. Bialosky JE, Bishop MD, Price DD, Robinson ME and George SZ (2009). The mechanisms of manual therapy in the treatment of

musculoskeletal pain: A comprehensive model. Manual Therapy, 14(5), 531–538. ↑

16. Lohr GA, O'Brien JC, Nodine DL and Brennan PC (1990). Natural killer cells as an outcome of chiropractic treatment efficacy. In Proceedings of the International Conference on Spinal Manipulation (pp. 109–112). Arlington, VA: Foundation for Chiropractic Education and Research. ↑
17. Haavik-Taylor H and Murphy B (2007). Cervical spine manipulation alters sensorimotor integration: A somatosensory evoked potential study. Clinical Neurophysiology, 118(2), 391–402. ↑
18. Milbocker KA, Smith IF and Klintsova AY (2024). Maintaining a dynamic brain: A review of empirical findings describing the roles of exercise, learning, and environmental enrichment in neuroplasticity from 2017–2023. Brain Plasticity, 9(1–2), 1–31. ↑
19. Lelic D, Niazi IK, Holt K, Jochumsen M, et al (2016). Manipulation of dysfunctional spinal joints affects sensorimotor integration in the prefrontal cortex: A brain source localization study. Neural Plasticity, 2016, Article 3704964. ↑
20. Roffers S, Huber L, Morris D, Stiles A, Barton D, House T. A randomized controlled trial to measure the effects of specific thoracic chiropractic adjustments on blood pressure and pulse rate. Clin Chiropr. 2011;14:169–70. ↑
21. Roffers S, Stiles A, Huber L, Morris D, Barton D, House T. Measuring the effects of specific cervical chiropractic adjustments on blood pressure and pulse rate: A randomized controlled trial. Clin Chiropr. 2011;4:170. ↑
22. Haas A, Chung J, Kent C, Mills B, McCoy M. Vertebral Subluxation and Systems Biology: An Integrative Review Exploring the Salutogenic Influence of Chiropractic Care on the Neuroendocrine-Immune System. Cureus. 2024 Mar 15;16(3):e56223. ↑

23. Sampath KK, Tumilty S, Wooten L, Belcher S, Farrell G and Gisselman AS (2024). Effectiveness of spinal manipulation in influencing the autonomic nervous system: A systematic review and meta-analysis. Journal of Manual & Manipulative Therapy, 32(1), 10–27. ↑
24. Tuchin PJ (1998). The effect of chiropractic spinal manipulative therapy on salivary cortisol levels. Chiropractic & Osteopathy, 7(2), 86–92. ↑
25. Chang AM, Aeschbach D, Duffy and Czeisler CA (2015). Evening use of light-emitting eReaders negatively affects sleep, circadian timing, and next-morning alertness. Proceedings of the National Academy of Sciences, 112(4), 1232–1237. ↑
26. Porges SW (2009). The polyvagal theory: New insights into adaptive reactions of the autonomic nervous system. Cleveland Clinic Journal of Medicine, 76(Suppl. 2), S86–S90. ↑
27. Hébert JJ, Stomski NJ, French SD and Rubinstein SM (2013). Serious adverse events and spinal manipulative therapy of the low back region: A systematic review of cases. Journal of Manipulative and Physiological Therapeutics, 36(9), 621–633. ↑
28. Kranenburg HA, Schmitt MA, Puentedura EJ, Luijckx GJ and Van der Schans CP (2017). Adverse events associated with the use of cervical spine manipulation or mobilization and patient characteristics: A systematic review. Musculoskeletal Science and Practice, 28, 32–38. ↑
29. Cassidy JD, Boyle E, Côté P, He Y, Hogg-Johnson S, Silver FL and Bondy SJ (2008). Risk of vertebrobasilar stroke and chiropractic care: Results of a population-based case-control and case-crossover study. Spine, 33(4 Suppl.), S176–S183. ↑
30. Nielsen SM, Tarp S, Christensen R, Bliddal H, Klokker L and Henriksen M (2017). The risk associated with spinal manipulation:

An overview of reviews. Systematic Reviews, 6, 64. ↑

31. Holt KR, Niazi IK, Johnson MI et al. (2016). Effectiveness of chiropractic care to improve sensorimotor function associated with falls risk in older people: A randomized controlled trial. Journal of Manipulative and Physiological Therapeutics, 39(4), 267–278. ↑
32. Lisi AJ, Wayne PM, Hausdorff JM et al. (2022). A systematic review of chiropractic care for fall prevention: Rationale, state of the evidence, and recommendations for future research. BMC Musculoskeletal Disorders, 23, 746. ↑
33. Billy GG, Lemieux SK and Chow MX (2014). Changes in lumbar disk morphology associated with prolonged sitting assessed by magnetic resonance imaging. PM&R, 6(9), 790–795. ↑
34. Wong AYL, Chan TPM, Chau AWM, Cheung HT, Kwan KCK, Lam AKH, Wong PYC and De Carvalho D (2019). Do different sitting postures affect spinal biomechanics of asymptomatic individuals? Gait & Posture, 67, 230–235. ↑

About the Author

Dr. Steven D. Roffers, DC is a licensed Doctor of Chiropractic with 38 years of experience in healthcare, biomedical science, rehabilitation, and clinical research. His diverse professional background uniquely positions him to explain both the science and philosophy of chiropractic care to a broad audience.

Dr. Roffers earned his Doctor of Chiropractic degree from Life University, graduating with scholastic honors and receiving the institution's prestigious *Clinic Excellence Award*. He was also a research scholarship recipient in the university's Office of Sponsored Research and Scholarly Activity and served on the faculty prior to entering private practice.

Dr. Roffers has contributed to numerous scientific publications and collaborated with investigators associated with organizations such as the Centers for Disease Control and Prevention and the National Cancer Institute. His research experience provides a rigorous foundation in evidence-based medicine and scientific inquiry that continues to inform his clinical work today.

Dr. Roffers has authored, edited, and reviewed medical books, white papers, and peer-reviewed journal articles and has served and continues to serve on multiple editorial boards. He is also the Director of the Chiropractic Research Alliance which is a professional group of 8,400+ chiropractors from across the world.

Life Is Better Adjusted represents the culmination of Dr. Roffers' lifelong commitment to understanding the relationship between structure, function, nervous system regulation, and human health and longevity.